Hay Fever

Dr Paul Carson is a member of the British Society for Allergy and Clinical Immunology, and the European Academy of Allergology and Clinical Immunology. He is a board member of the Irish Lung Foundation and an advisory member of the Severe Asthma Advisory Group in Ireland. He has written several other self-help books for adults and children on allergy-related topics, including *Sinusitis: Steps to healing* (Sheldon Press, 2009). <www.allergy-ireland.ie>

Overcoming Common Problems Series

Selected titles

A full list of titles is available from Sheldon Press,
36 Causton Street, London SW1P 4ST and on our website at
www.sheldonpress.co.uk

101 Questions to Ask Your Doctor
Dr Tom Smith

Asperger Syndrome in Adults
Dr Ruth Searle

The Assertiveness Handbook
Mary Hartley

Assertiveness: Step by step
Dr Windy Dryden and Daniel Constantinou

Backache: What you need to know
Dr David Delvin

Birth Over 35
Sheila Kitzinger

Body Language: What you need to know
David Cohen

Bulimia, Binge-eating and their Treatment
Professor J. Hubert Lacey, Dr Bryony Bamford
and Amy Brown

The Cancer Survivor's Handbook
Dr Terry Priestman

The Chronic Pain Diet Book
Neville Shone

Cider Vinegar
Margaret Hills

Coeliac Disease: What you need to know
Alex Gazzola

**Coping Successfully with Chronic Illness:
Your healing plan**
Neville Shone

Coping Successfully with Pain
Neville Shone

Coping Successfully with Prostate Cancer
Dr Tom Smith

Coping Successfully with Shyness
Margaret Oakes, Professor Robert Bor
and Dr Carina Eriksen

Coping Successfully with Ulcerative Colitis
Peter Cartwright

Coping Successfully with Varicose Veins
Christine Craggs-Hinton

Coping Successfully with Your Hiatus Hernia
Dr Tom Smith

Coping When Your Child Has Cerebral Palsy
Jill Eckersley

Coping with Anaemia
Dr Tom Smith

Coping with Asthma in Adults
Mark Greener

**Coping with Birth Trauma and Postnatal
Depression**
Lucy Jolin

Coping with Bowel Cancer
Dr Tom Smith

Coping with Bronchitis and Emphysema
Dr Tom Smith

Coping with Candida
Shirley Trickett

Coping with Chemotherapy
Dr Terry Priestman

Coping with Chronic Fatigue
Trudie Chalder

Coping with Coeliac Disease
Karen Brody

Coping with Diverticulitis
Peter Cartwright

Coping with Drug Problems in the Family
Lucy Jolin

Coping with Dyspraxia
Jill Eckersley

Coping with Early-onset Dementia
Jill Eckersley

**Coping with Eating Disorders
and Body Image**
Christine Craggs-Hinton

Coping with Envy
Dr Windy Dryden

Coping with Gout
Christine Craggs-Hinton

Coping with Headaches and Migraine
Alison Frith

Coping with Heartburn and Reflux
Dr Tom Smith

Coping with Life after Stroke
Dr Mareeni Raymond

**Coping with Life's Challenges: Moving on
from adversity**
Dr Windy Dryden

Overcoming Common Problems Series

Overcoming Common Problems Series

Overcoming Common Problems

Hay Fever
How to beat it

DR PAUL CARSON

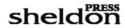

First published in Great Britain in 2013

Sheldon Press
36 Causton Street
London SW1P 4ST
www.sheldonpress.co.uk

British Library Cataloguing-in-Publication Data
A catalogue record for this book is available from the British Library

ISBN 978–1–84709–283–0
eBook ISBN 978–1–84709–284–7

Typeset by Fakenham Prepress Solutions, Fakenham, Norfolk NR21 8NN
First printed in Great Britain by Ashford Colour Press
Subsequently digitally printed in Great Britain

eBook by Fakenham Prepress Solutions, Fakenham, Norfolk NR21 8NN

Produced on paper from sustainable forests

Contents

Introduction

Aaaacccchhhhooooo! It's that time of year again. 'Get me a tissue quick.' *Aaaacccchhhhooooo!* 'For goodness sake pass the tissues.' *Aaaacccchhhhooooo!* 'I wish it would rain. I hate this weather.'

Yes, you're having yet another summer sneezing bout. Maybe the winter wasn't especially harsh and spring dragged on longer than usual, but now the warm weather has arrived and there seems to be a bounce to everyone's step. The nights are shorter, the days longer, with glorious blue skies and a big yellow sun to enjoy. Neighbours haul out barbecues and prepare for lazy outdoor evenings. Newspapers feature gardening supplements and the sound of lawn mowers drowns the drone of traffic. These are wonderful, relaxing conditions for most people, but not for you. You dread even putting your nose outside the back window. You've been laid low for yet another summer with what seems like the worst head cold ever. You've got hay fever and little sympathy.

'It's only a nose allergy,' mumbles your doctor as he scribbles a prescription for an antihistamine that you could have bought over the counter anyway. 'Anyway, it'll go when it rains,' he adds by way of dismissal.

Sniff, snuffle, sneeze and out you go, totally disillusioned.

You search the internet and find a bagful of offers:

Hay fever, read about our natural cures.
Honey, the sweetest cure for hay fever.
Ten of the best hay fever remedies.
How to cure yourself of hay fever . . . we will tell you how to cure hay fever yourself.

It all sounds great, but secretly you suspect it might not be true. If there's a cure for hay fever why isn't everyone using it?

On a positive note your chemist is very helpful. He explains the array of products he assures you will help. Homeopathy, natural oils, local honey and the same pharmaceutical items you've seen promoted on TV and read about in magazines. But you tried them last year and they didn't work. And your friends tried them too and few found them helpful.

What *are* you going to do?

Aaaaccchhhhoooo! There you go again, grabbing the tissue box and trying to stop mascara running down your face. You feel awful. Exhausted and getting only fitful sleep.

Don't panic. Using flexible fibre optics to observe the state of the nose lining in real time has given doctors new insights into the condition. We now know hay fever affects the sinuses as well as the nose. It triggers eye problems and 'chestiness' and brings on a sense of fatigue that is often overwhelming. But better strategies offer hay fever patients the chance to recover their lives and enjoy summers like other folk.

Aaaaccchhhhoooo! Stop preaching and tell me, what's the right treatment?

Don't be so impatient, I know the answers. I've been dealing with allergy problems for almost 30 years and I have the inside track on hay fever. I know how it affects people and why it's so disabling. Treating it as nothing more than a nuisance leaves sufferers miserable and prone to other conditions such as asthma.

So put away that box of tissues. There is a plan for everybody, including you.

This book will take you through all remedies, conventional and unorthodox, and gently tease you along the correct path to good health.

Please don't jump straight to the chapter on treatments. Take time to read how your nose works and what happens when it stops working. Being informed allows you to understand the therapies better.

So turn the page and read. And start enjoying life again.

1

What is hay fever and why does it make me feel miserable?

Simply put, hay fever is mainly an allergic reaction to grass pollen. If that was the beginning and end of it, you wouldn't feel so miserable each summer. Nor would it seem so difficult to manage. Let's put the easy terms aside, though, and focus on what really happens. Because hay fever is a far from simple problem. For some it's a nightmare.

It *is* an aggressive allergic reaction to pollen grains (10,000 grass pollen grains would fit on the tip of a needle). But it's what happens to the person who has hay fever – which until recently has been poorly understood – that makes it so difficult to manage. And sheer misery for the patient.

What causes hay fever?

Hay fever is a particularly seasonal (especially midsummer) problem, but can start earlier and even drag on into early autumn. It's caused by the tiny pollen grains, about one millionth of an inch across, that are released by trees and shrubs and flowering plants in spring and by grass in summer. They are essentially tiny bundles of DNA, each enclosed in a tough protein coat that protects the precious genetic material. This protein coat can – in some people – trigger a violent allergic reaction. The substance causing the reaction, in this case grass pollen, is called an *allergen*. It seems to cause the body's immune system to mount an attack, as if it were being invaded by harmful bacteria or viruses. The body releases histamine (one of the main chemicals involved in allergic reactions) into the bloodstream, and this causes the inflammation in the sinuses, eyes and airways. There's a more detailed explanation of allergy in Chapter 6.

Allowing for weather variations, the pollen season starts in the south of Europe. In the UK and Ireland aggressive sneezes can be heard first along the warmer western coasts. By the end of May high pollen counts can be detected countrywide (the pollen count measures the amount of pollen in the air over 24 hours). High levels of pollen occur on warm, dry and sunny days. Low levels occur on wet, damp and cold days. Rain washes pollen out of the air. Pollen is released in the morning and carried higher into the air by midday. It descends again to 'nose level' in the late afternoon. Cities and dense urban areas stay warmer longer and hold pollen. Combine this with atmospheric pollution from car fumes and you can understand why city dwellers suffer more aggressive hay fever than their country cousins.

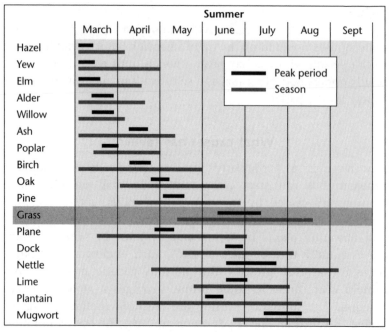

Figure 1.1 Which pollens cause your allergy?

On the calendar, highlight the months when your hay fever occurs. See when it coincides with the plant pollen pattern to work out which pollens you're allergic to. Grass pollen is the commonest cause of hay fever between May and July.

Only the general pattern of pollen production in the UK is shown. Depending on the weather and region, the timing and severity will vary.

So what's new that makes me confident hay fever can be beaten? New drugs? New nose clips and sunglasses? Glass bubbles that fit over the head and filter the air we breathe during the pollen season? No, more important and simpler than that. Doctors now know exactly what happens inside the nose during an allergy attack. And they know (at long last) how to reverse it.

Read on.

Investigating symptoms using fibre-optic technology

Recently doctors have found flexible fibre-optics vital in their understanding of nose, sinus, throat and vocal cord disorders. No more than a narrow tube covered in protective sealed plastic with a camera chip at the tip, these devices allow enlarged and dramatic images to be obtained. This, in turn, allows us to grasp what's going wrong in the tissue being observed.

A fibrescope – a flexible fibre-optic tube with camera chip attached (see Figure 1.2) – is inserted into the nose and threaded all

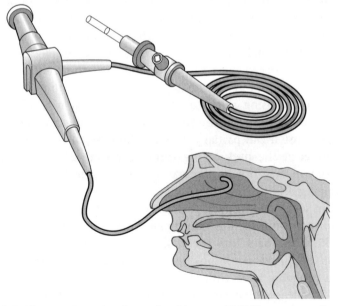

Figure 1.2 Fibre-optic technology: the Olympus ENF fibrescope – for easy observation and diagnosis

the way to the vocal cords. The fibrescope is no more than 3 mm in diameter, so it passes easily and painlessly. The state of the nose and all structures within the nose can be seen and recorded. The sinus openings can be observed. The usefulness of this instrument cannot be underestimated, as it allows the treating doctor to have a better understanding of what the patient is complaining about, and the likely causes.

Modern flexible fibre-optic technology used during an attack of hay fever shows dramatic swelling of the delicate membrane that lines the nose – so you get a blocked nose. The lining also becomes extremely irritable, making you sneeze. It secretes mucus, giving you a runny nose, with the result that you use boxes of tissues like there's no tomorrow. Fibre optics also show how the narrow openings into the sinuses (see below) become totally blocked, causing sinus pain and congestion – that dull ache you feel along the forehead and cheek bones.

And as the allergic challenge (the invasion of pollen grains into the nose) progresses, extra swelling occurs in the upper part of the nose. This squeezes the nerve ending for taste and smells located there and soon it ceases to function. So severely troubled hay fever sufferers may lose their senses of taste and smell, important quality of life sensations. You mightn't notice you've left the gas on. Flick a switch and suddenly you've got third degree burns as well as a blocked nose. Or you might miss the scent of summer rose blooms. Or notice that your food tastes quite bland, and that you're using more salt than is good just to get a taste of what you're eating. If the nasal obstruction progresses beyond the upper nose it can partially obstruct the Eustachian tube, a narrow channel at the back of the throat connecting to the inner ear. Now you may not hear properly, and get a feeling your ears are popping.

Are you nodding 'yes' to most of these? Let me throw in that unpleasant mucus flow that trickles down the back of your throat, making you hack into the sink or spit into tissues at work when (you hope) no one's looking. Doctors call this 'post-nasal drip'. You probably have your own name for it. Almost certainly your work colleagues have a secret phrase they bandy about at the water cooler. Most are not repeatable in polite company.

Next, there's yet another nerve ending that links the nose and sinuses to the lungs (explained in detail in Chapter 3), so that hay fever can make you cough, wheeze and feel short of breath. In fact it can trigger asthma for the first time, or worsen pre-existing asthma so you may use your inhalers more than usual. Then (believe it or not) there is a final nerve ending (or reflex, called the naso-ocular reflex) that links the inner lining of the nose to the outer surface of the eyes. When that nerve becomes irritated the eyes redden, itch, water and swell. As pollen grains come into direct contact with the eye lining, the redness, itching and swelling worsens and the skin around the eyes fills with fluid, making them look puffy. In very severe hay fever, especially with children, the lining of the eye can be damaged from constant rubbing for relief from the intense itch. And the inner surface of the upper lids (in particular) swell with what look like 'cobblestone' bumps. These bumps irritate the delicate eye surface further, causing more discomfort. More importantly, they can cause eye damage and must be dealt with by an eye specialist.

I'm not finished (stop groaning). Some folk with hay fever notice that the inside of their mouth, lips and tongue itch and swell slightly when they eat certain fruits during the pollen season. This is known as the 'oral-allergy syndrome'. Here the protein in certain foods cross-reacts with the airborne pollen grains that you're allergic to. This triggers itching and slight swelling of the lips, tongue and back of the throat. For example, if you're allergic to birch tree pollen you may also react to celery, curry spices, raw tomato, raw carrot, apples, pears and kiwi fruit. If you're allergic to grass pollen you may react to oats, rye, wheat, kiwi fruit and raw tomato. If your allergy is to weed pollen, you may again react to raw carrot and curry spices.

Put all that in a package and you now understand the word *suffer*. And grasp the concept *miserable*. Hay fever victims are swamped with the combined symptoms of a runny, itchy and blocked nose (the medical term is *allergic rhinitis*); partially blocked ears with reduced hearing (*serous otitis media*); impaired senses of taste and smell (*anosmia*); cough and wheezing (*allergic asthma*); and red, itchy, swollen eyes (*allergic conjunctivitis*). And, because it also blocks the sinus openings, it makes you feel totally drained (non-medical terms include whacked, drained, worn out, exhausted, fed up and want-to-curl-up-in-a-ball-and-die).

Symptom summary

In case you don't know them all too well already, these are the main symptoms of hay fever:

- sneezing;
- a blocked and runny nose;
- sinus congestion with headaches, especially along the forehead;
- itchy, red and watery eyes;
- puffy eyes and lower eyelids;
- a cough and occasional wheezing;
- ears popping, and occasional hearing impairment;
- diminished senses of taste and smell (in those with severe hay fever);
- an itch along the roof of the mouth and the back of the throat when eating certain foods;
- a feeling of intense lethargy.

The sinuses

Sinuses are cave-like pockets in the skull. They run alongside the nose and connect directly to it via small tubes. If the nose becomes inflamed, the sinuses soon become involved as well. The functions of sinuses include humidifying air, providing cushioning for the skull and increasing the resonance of the voice.

There are four types of sinuses that surround the nose (see Figures 1.3 to 1.6); they're called the *maxillary*, *frontal*, *sphenoid* and *ethmoid* sinuses. When each (or all) is inflamed from allergic challenge, you may experience many different symptoms.

So why does this all start in the first place? Because you're allergic. And your allergy is to the pollen grains carried in the air during the warmer spring and summer months. Most people are troubled by grass pollen only, but a significant number are caught with the combined curse of tree pollen allergy as well as grass pollen allergy. So their season starts in early spring with mild hay fever symptoms.

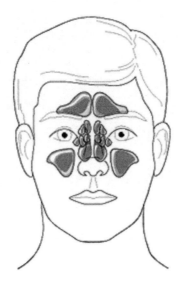

Figure 1.3 The sinuses

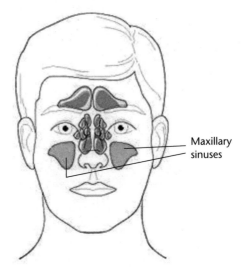

Maxillary
sinuses

Figure 1.4 The maxillary sinuses

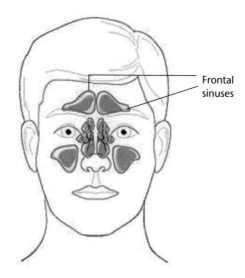

Figure 1.5 The frontal sinuses

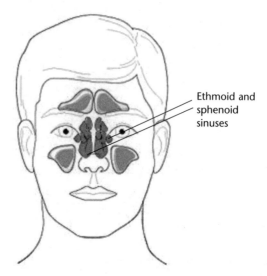

Figure 1.6 The ethmoid and sphenoid sinuses

By the time the grass pollen months arrive they are already compromised, so that even small amounts of grass pollen can trigger quite aggressive hay fever. If the summer is especially warm and sunny with high surges of pollen, then those three to four months can be a write-off.

Thankfully, help is at hand. But before we discuss treatments, the following self-help tips are worth considering.

- Avoid areas of lush grassland.
- Keep house and car windows closed during the peak pollen hours of late morning and late afternoon.
- Wear wraparound sunglasses to reduce pollen grains affecting the eyes.
- If you can, avoid being outdoors in the late morning and late afternoon.
- Don't smoke and keep away from smokers (passive smoking aggravates all allergies).
- Get someone else to mow the lawn or wear a face mask if you have to cut the grass.
- Choose seaside breaks for holidays as offshore breezes blow pollen away.
- Check TV, radio and newspapers for the next day's pollen count and plan your schedule accordingly.
- Put a smear of Vaseline inside each nostril to ease the soreness and to capture pollen entering the nasal passages.
- Never sleep with the bedroom window open.
- Put used tea bags in the fridge. They make great soothing compresses to relieve swollen or puffy eyes.
- Keep an antihistamine handy for sudden allergy attacks (this does not contradict the advice you'll read in Chapter 4).
- Remember to think about the foods you eat and which may react with the pollen you're allergic to (oral-allergy syndrome). In particular be careful of celery, curry spices, raw tomato, raw carrot, apples, pears, kiwi fruit, oats, rye and wheat.

Would it be better if I moved to another country?

Not really, and let me explain why. I lived and worked in Australia between 1977 and 1982. While there I dealt with many patients from Britain and Ireland who'd emigrated in the sixties and seventies 'for health reasons'. Many had been advised to move to a warmer climate to help their recurring chest problems. In those days it was described as bronchitis (implying chest infections). In reality it was allergic asthma, with its associated nose and sinus problems. Moving to Australia did offer immediate (but short-term) relief. Most of these 'chesty' and 'nasal' adults and children became very well for the first time in their lives. The constant head colds and coughs abated, the winters spent with their heads over hot bowls of eucalyptus ended. They noticed dramatic improvements in their quality of life. Why? Because they'd put considerable distance between themselves and the environment in which they grew up (which they were allergic to). So the heavy curtains and carpets for warmth and closed windows to save heat used in Northern European countries – havens for dust mites, another common cause of allergies (see Chapter 6) – were replaced with tiled floors and open windows. Feeling cold was no longer an issue. British and Irish native pollens didn't fill the Australian air in that country's summer.

Unfortunately the improvements didn't last. These folk, in time, became allergic to the native Australian environment. Within three to five years they were as bad (indeed, sometimes worse) than they remembered back home.

So, in answer to the query 'Shouldn't I just move to another country?' the disappointing response is 'no'. You take your 'allergicness' with you wherever you travel. Stay in one place long enough and you soon become sensitized to that location, and the same old allergy issues of blocked noses, aching sinuses and wheezy chests surface. The best long-term therapy is immunotherapy (see Chapter 5), where doctors use a strategy to calm down 'allergicness' rather than have you desperately try to change the world around you. Despite your understandable frustration, you can't chop down every tree and concrete over every grassy verge and garden in your neighbourhood.

Finally, there is a group of allergy sufferers who have an all-year-round 'hay fever' that becomes dramatically worse in the summer. They usually have an additional dust mite or animal hair sensitivity that keeps the nose and sinus tissue constantly inflamed. Along comes a warm, sunny day with high levels of pollen in the air and suddenly their nose and sinuses become totally obstructed. They feel miserable, tired and exhausted. They have sinus congestion, itchy and red eyes and often wheezy chests. Old patches of healed eczema become irritable again and the urge to scratch becomes too much. What was once healthy skin now becomes dry, red and inflamed.

If your head has nearly nodded off your shoulders (or you recognize much of this in your child) agreeing with what I've described, don't panic. There is so much your doctor can do to help that you need never suffer such misery again. Next we'll look at all-year-round hay fever.

2

All-year-round hay fever

Many patients attending my clinic wonder if they have hay fever all year round. Sure, their obvious hay fever symptoms worsen during high pollen months. But, expecting everything to improve by autumn, they find that their horribly stuffy nose stubbornly stays blocked. Their tissue use doesn't decrease and they feel almost as bad as they remembered feeling at the height of the pollen season. And other niggling issues are becoming obvious. Dull headaches, especially along the forehead. A diminished sense of smell, and possibly of taste. Coughing more than usual and getting puffed out with even slight exercise. Here the problem is no longer hay fever (though that may have been the trigger at the beginning); rather these folk are troubled with all-year-round rhinitis (nasal inflammation – swelling and irritability of the tissues involved).

The nose lining connects directly with the sinuses, so the condition quickly progresses from a nose-only complaint to a nose-plus-sinus issue. The usual reason for this all-year-round hay fever (which doctors call *perennial rhinitis*) is a combination of allergic responses to the environment. All-year-round hay fever is almost always the end result of allergy to dust mites (read more on this in Chapter 6) or possibly to animal hair, plus tree pollens, plus grass pollens. These sufferers don't stand a chance. They stagger through the winter challenges of dust mite or animal hair allergy that obstructs and irritates their noses. Then, just when they should be getting relief from a more outdoor lifestyle, they walk straight into the tree pollen and grass pollen seasons. Before they know it they're suffering more than ever before. By the time they call on me for help they almost always have a degree of sinusitis (inflammation of the sinus tissue) as well, and nose blockage.

All-year-round hay fever tends to provoke particularly aggressive symptoms, including occasional infection with fever, green or yellow nasal discharge, blurred vision and intense headache. All-year-round hay fever is complicated because there may be a number of interrelated causes. Doctors use a big word for this (doctors like using big words and strange-sounding names . . . it makes us feel important): *multi-factorial*. In plain English this suggests there may be a number of different triggers coming together at the same time to cause chaos. This is the perfect storm of nose and sinus problems. Allergy testing, blood testing, a certain type of X-ray called a CT scan, nasal endoscopies and acid reflux studies (explained later in this chapter) are often used to clarify the situation.

The simple questionnaire (right) will indicate if you may have a nasal allergy.

Jennifer

Jennifer is a 38-year-old public health nurse. For the past 12 months she's been feeling sluggish, tired and lethargic a lot of the time. She has a constant headache that has become more of a nuisance in the past few months. She rarely wakens feeling refreshed and has to be careful not to nod off driving the car.

A nursing colleague wonders out loud at the amount of tissues making Jennifer's handbag bulge. 'You must have hay fever,' she offers. But it's snowing outside, with not as much as one pollen grain floating in the air. 'Well, that head cold you have has been dragging on for months now.'

Jennifer's colleague's observation prompts her to make an appointment with her family doctor. 'Can you get hay fever in the winter?' she asks. His puzzled expression is the only answer and Jennifer suspects there's something else going on.

When the doctor inspects the internal lining of Jennifer's nose he notices that the membrane is so swollen it's obstructing her ability to breathe freely. He suspects Jennifer cannot get a refreshing night's sleep because of this and suggests the explanation for her symptoms is not all-year-round hay fever, but rather that she has a persisting perennial rhinitis with probable sinus involvement. Jennifer is astonished; she never thought of herself as a sinus sufferer. 'What's causing this?' she asks. A battery of tests and sinus scans are arranged to answer Jennifer's understandable question.

The scan shows considerable thickening of the sinuses on Jennifer's forehead (the frontal sinuses; see Figure 1.5 on page 8) as well as those to the sides of her nose (maxillary and ethmoid; Figures 1.4 and 1.6 on pages 7 and 8). The scan also confirms the doctor's observation about swelling of the nasal membrane.

Allergy testing shows Jennifer has a cat allergy (she has two tabbies

Over 12 months, how many of these symptoms do you get?

- Itchy nose
- runny nose
- blocked nose
- sneezing fits
- a dull headache along the forehead
- a dulled sense of smell
- itchy eyes
- watery eyes.

Score 2 points for every 'yes'. If your total score is 6 or above then you probably have some type of nasal allergy that could include hay fever.

Do you feel especially worse

- in spring
- in summer
- in the countryside
- near animals such as cats or dogs or horses
- when in bed
- in rooms with heavy curtains and thick pile carpets
- when you eat particular foods?

When you get these symptoms, how unwell do you feel on a scale of 1 to 10 (if 1 is feeling perfectly normal and 10 is feeling absolutely miserable and drained of all energy)?

- If your symptom score is 5 or over, especially if they are linked to the spring and summer seasons and you notice an obvious link to being in the countryside, then you probably have a pollen allergy. If you notice food-related symptoms, then – BINGO – it's a pollen allergy.
- If your symptoms link to being near animals only, then you almost certainly have an animal hair allergy. Worse in rooms with heavy curtains and thick pile carpets? Probably a dust mite allergy.

that are long-haired; they roam her apartment as if they own the place). She also has a strong dust mite allergy – and a grass pollen allergy, though this is not as important as her cat and dust mite sensitivity.

Jennifer has to make some difficult choices. Does she take a lot of medication to reduce the swelling in her nose and sinuses and live with the cats? Or does she do the more sensible and logical thing: get rid of the cats and do a cleaning blitz in her apartment to eradicate all traces of cat hair and dust mites? 'Do nothing and I suspect you'll eventually develop asthma,' warns her doctor. 'Then we won't be discussing the cats, we'll be talking about which inhaler you need to use and what to do if you get an asthma attack.' The argument is won, if reluctantly. The cats find new homes and Jennifer employs a specialist cleaning firm to 'de-allergy' her apartment. She also takes some prescribed medicine to help while the clean-up progresses.

Within three months her quality of life dramatically improves and she feels reinvigorated. She's saving a fortune on paper tissues and cat food. Six months later a follow-up sinus scan shows almost total clearance of the swollen lining inside the sinuses and nose. Of course she misses her tabbies. Of course she hates vacuuming the apartment. But compared to the significantly impaired quality of life she was experiencing, the trade-off is worth it.

Other causes of all-year-round hay fever

All-year-round hay fever is not always an allergy issue alone. Quite often there are a number of interrelated factors involved.

- Allergy, as described earlier, and usually to inhaled allergy-provoking substances such as dust mites, pollens, animal hair, etc..
- Cigarette smoking.
- Environmental irritants such as cement dust, laboratory fumes, ammonia dyes in hairdressing salons, etc..
- Atmospheric pollution.
- Poor air conditioning in your workplace.
- Over-use of nasal decongestants.
- Hormone changes in women. The menopause causes significant nose and sinus irritability. So too can the oral contraceptive pill and hormone replacement therapy.
- Structural defects that you might have been born with or acquired. These include abnormally narrow nose-to-sinus chan-

nels (you're born with these) or a bent nose due to the central cartilage in the nose, called the nasal septum, being crooked. You may have had this since childhood or acquired it through injury. If a structural defect is causing your problems, then only corrective surgery will allow you lead a normal life. All the drugs in the world won't work: a surgical cure is vital.

- Cocaine abuse. This is an increasing problem for doctors dealing with hay fever. Cocaine wears away the nasal lining and may even destroy the bony cartilage that separates one nostril from the other. Cocaine users have overly exaggerated symptoms. They complain bitterly about the pain and malaise of their hay fever, the dramatic discomfort they experience and that 'nothing I've been given helps'. Nothing will help (or can help) while the cocaine abuse continues. Unfortunately, people who frequently use cocaine have little grasp of the connection between their poor health and drug addiction. They deny any link when it's pointed out. 'I haven't done coke for a month and my hay fever is just as bad,' they say – an attitude that tries the patience of many doctors.

Gerry
Gerry is a successful accountant. He earns good money, is single and lives in an apartment. He likes the good life and is a 'recreational' drug user. His favourite night out is a few beers in the pub, wine with an Indian or Chinese meal and then off to a nightclub to party. He'll probably smoke a few joints en route and snort cocaine in the toilets. He may even take an 'E' to keep the party mood flowing. However Gerry's behaviour is becoming increasingly erratic, he's prone to mood swings, is easily angered and seems to have recurring hay fever. He complains bitterly that his GP can't do anything for him and even an ear, nose and throat specialist was 'useless'. Inevitably Gerry's lifestyle catches up with him: after a heavy night of drink and drugs he falls, bangs his head and is taken to A&E. He is semi-conscious and disorientated, his speech slurred, so the doctors decide to keep him in for investigation. They fear he has suffered a serious head injury. Blood tests reveal high levels of alcohol, amphetamines and cocaine. Scans show no injury to the brain but considerable damage to the nose and sinuses. Gerry is referred to a rehab unit but fails to keep his appointment. Gerry will party until he drops dead or throws himself off a height believing he can fly. The UK and Ireland have plenty of Gerrys and the number is growing.

How do doctors find out which triggers cause all-year-round hay fever?

Commonly doctors answer this question on the basis of how the symptoms began (called 'the history'). They will ask some of the following questions to get more information.

- How long is it since you were last fully well?
- How did this so-called hay fever start, slowly or suddenly?
- Do you have any ideas what brought it on in the first place or makes it worse now?
- What have you found helpful in giving you relief so far?
- What have you tried that didn't make any difference or, even, made you feel worse?
- Have you been using a lot of non-prescription nasal decongestants?
- How is your general health?
- Do you have any background medical condition that may be irritating your nose and sinuses?
- Do you snore?
- Do you mouth breathe while asleep?
- Do you get a lot of post-nasal drip?
- Do you suffer heartburn?
- Is your sense of smell or taste impaired?
- Do you have asthma or do you get 'chesty' each time your sinuses act up?

The answers to these give valuable insight into the type of sinus problem you may have.

Next there is a general physical examination to make sure the hay fever isn't but one of a group of features of certain conditions.

In most specialist hay fever centres an allergy test is now performed. This is usually done by means of the 'skin-prick test' format, described in more detail in Chapter 6. With a skin-prick test the doctor places a concentrated drop of allergy extract onto the skin. Each drop contains a test substance such as dust mite, cat hair, horsehair, grass pollen or a specific food.

The test drop is brought into direct contact with the skin mast cells by pricking the surface and allowing the fluid to seep to a lower level. The mast cells hold the body's memory for allergy, in other words they recognize what you are allergic to.

If you are allergic to a specific substance, there will be a visible reaction. The size of the central blister, plus any surrounding skin redness, tells the doctor what you are allergic to and how strongly allergic.

The final interpretation depends on symptoms, what the doctor discovers when he examines your nose and what reactions come up on testing.

Probably a range of blood tests will be arranged at this point to check your general health and offer insights into any background ailments that might produce hay fever-type symptoms. For example, immune disorders, including the inability to manufacture the cells that fight infection (antibodies), are occasionally a cause of persisting all-year-round hay fever. The final interpretation can include monitoring your body's ability to make antibodies after vaccination. Some centres treat patients with reduced immunity with intravenous gamma-globulin antibody therapy. This is an infusion by drip of specific immune cells to boost immunity and increase the ability to fight infection.

These tests are followed by direct inspection of the nose, possibly using a simple light source (much the same sort of instrument that doctors use to look in patients' ears). However this gives only a limited view of the nose and sinuses. More commonly a flexible fibre-optic tool such as the Olympus ENF fibrescope (as shown in Figure 1.2 on page 3) with camera chip attached is inserted into the nose and threaded all the way to the vocal cords. The usefulness of this instrument cannot be underestimated as it allows the treating doctor to have a better understanding of what the patient is complaining about and the likely causes.

A certain type of X-ray called a CT scan may be ordered to give a clearer picture of what's happening in the sinuses. CT scans highlight the soft membranes of the nose and sinuses and show allergic changes or infection. There is a significant amount of radiology exposure with CT scan imaging, so don't expect your treating doctor to order this at the drop of a tissue. Also, these scans are expensive and healthcare budgetary restraints may dictate that they are to be reserved only for very ill patients.

Finally, where there is any suspicion of stomach acid reflux (if you answered 'yes' to the heartburn question), an evaluation of the stomach and gullet may be ordered. This may take the form of a gastroscopy (a flexible fibre-optic device, passed directly into the stomach via the gullet) or a barium-swallow X-ray. Here a radio-active dye (barium) is swallowed and its passage through the gullet and stomach captured on X-ray. This may show significant spilling-back of stomach acid contents towards the nose and sinuses, irritating their delicate lining. Dietary changes plus anti-reflux drugs often cure this situation.

Post-nasal drip, without other symptoms of hay fever, is often caused by acid reflux.

Summary

With all-year-round hay fever your doctor will try to get to the bottom of all potential causes before selecting a treatment course. There's no point in shoving drugs at you until it is known whether or not there are any background triggers. Also, treatments are tai-lored to the cause. What might work for allergic hay fever will not make a blind bit of difference to infected sinusitis or a hormone-driven nasal obstruction. It may sound complicated, but in practice it's fairly straightforward.

3

How hay fever can trigger asthma

On 24 and 25 June 1994 London and the south-eastern counties of England experienced an asthma epidemic. This was associated with a thunderstorm and strong gusts of wind. It followed peak grass pollen concentrations in that part of Britain. Thousands of patients were affected, the numbers overwhelming hospitals and family doctors. The crisis didn't last long, maybe no more than a few hours. But those involved and who were subsequently tested showed they were very allergic to grass pollen. This (and similar events in Birmingham, as well as Melbourne in Australia and Barcelona in Spain) were researched in detail and many varying conclusions reached. Grass pollen surges seemed to be a major factor.

But, you say, grass pollen only causes hay fever. Doesn't it? Well, actually it causes a lot more than hay fever (bad as that is). If hay fever is aggressive it causes allergic inflammation of both the nose and the sinuses. The nose and sinuses are linked to the lungs by a number of pathways, as explained later in this chapter. So an aggressive attack of hay fever can trigger asthma. This is known in medical circles as *united airways disease* (and no, that's not a budget airline ailment!). United airways disease implies that asthma is but the lung component of a much more complicated condition that involves the nose, sinuses, lungs and bloodstream.

Elizabeth
Thirty-three-year-old publishing editor Elizabeth had an intractable cough. She also had asthma and was using standard full strength anti-asthma therapy. The cough was socially embarrassing and spoiled her quality of life. Any type of conversation was cut short by a bout of convulsive spluttering. Elizabeth attended two GPs in the same London practice and the respiratory unit of a top London teaching hospital. There she was reviewed by three specialists (one a pulmonary allergist) and had multiple tests including chest X-ray, pulmonary function tests and allergy tests. She showed very strong responses to dust

21

mites, pollens and cat hair. She was given a fact sheet on dust mites and de-cluttered her apartment to little more than bare boards and a wooden bed. Her cough continued. The hospital advised that nothing else could be done and suggested to her GP that this was possibly a psychological cough, recommending a mild tranquillizer. In desperation (and convinced it was not a psychological cough) Elizabeth sought help elsewhere.

During questioning at a reputable private allergy clinic, she agreed that her nose was blocked all the time, her senses of taste and smell were poor and her hearing had deteriorated ('I've had to turn up the volume on my iPod recently'). When examined she was found to have severe swelling of her nose lining. 'You're the first doctor to have inspected my nose,' she remarked. There was fluid behind both eardrums, suggesting Eustachian tube obstruction. Further questioning revealed she worked in a smoky office (the non-smoking ban hadn't come into effect in the UK in small offices) and its owner had a large cat that shed hair.

It was explained that the cough was almost certainly due to her aggressive, unrecognized and untreated nasal allergy. It was suggested that while her home environment might be perfect, her workplace was a definite health hazard. Elizabeth was treated appropriately and the nasal cavity stabilized. To say her life changed for the better is an understatement: symptom scores for her hay fever symptoms and asthma dropped by 80 per cent. The cough flared at work and in smoky environments, so she left her job and found a better (and safer) office. Now she is enjoying a dramatically improved lifestyle. Her hearing has improved as well. However she's quite annoyed with the NHS and that top London teaching hospital (not to mention her smoking colleagues and the boss's cat).

If an Oxford-educated (as Elizabeth is), articulate and successful publishing executive can have so much difficulty having her problem identified and treated, it says a lot about the continuing ignorance throughout the medical profession concerning the link between nose and sinus allergy and asthma. And its correct management.

Here are a few facts.

- Allergic hay fever may cause nasal symptoms only.
- Allergic hay fever often involves the sinuses as well as the nose.
- Allergic hay fever may provoke chest symptoms.
- Allergic hay fever may coexist with asthma.
- Children troubled with both asthma and allergic hay fever have more asthma-related hospital admissions than those children

with asthma alone (and no hay fever). They also spend more total days in hospital.

The relationship between allergic hay fever and asthma has been known for some time (though listening to some doctors you might find that hard to believe) and people commonly present with both disorders. Experts believe allergic hay fever and asthma are connected by a number of different pathways. For example, post-nasal drip may contain cells that slip into the lungs and trigger asthma-type symptoms. Also, blood units (called Th2) move from the nose and sinuses to the bone marrow to produce a number of allergy groupings. They then transfer into the blood and 'stick' in the nose, sinuses and lungs, causing further allergic inflammation. I appreciate that this is all very complicated and medical (and to be honest, I'm not sure I understand the half of it myself, but I do recognize the sense behind the theory). The bottom line is this: treat the affected nose and sinuses and you improve any coexisting asthma significantly.

All children with true asthma also have some type of nasal allergy. For example, when pollen-driven hay fever is active, lung tube irritability increases, often aggravating the symptoms of asthma. Furthermore, the onset of allergic hay fever sometimes precedes asthma, and the onset of summer asthma may be prevented by successful treatment of allergic hay fever.

Significant problems in the upper airways (i.e. the nose and sinuses) can produce symptoms in the lower respiratory tract (i.e. the lungs). Treat the upper respiratory problems and you can alleviate or even cure the lower respiratory trouble.

Harry

Harry is a 13-year-old with troublesome asthma. He's seen many doctors, including asthma specialists, and is on a lot of anti-asthma medication. But he's still troubled with his chest and each break-down in well-being seems to start during the hay fever season. There is a strong history of allergy in the family (two sisters had eczema as babies, his father suffers hay fever each summer) but no attention is paid to Harry's parents' request for allergy testing ('waste of time, could be anything, try lifting the carpets', are the dismissive comments). Each doctor advised that the boy had difficult asthma made worse by repeated virus infections. Live with it, they said. Stop annoying us, they didn't say but implied.

When Harry was evaluated at a reputable allergy centre a completely different interpretation was put on his ill-health and its management. The examining doctor inspected the inside lining of Harry's nose ('no other doctor has ever done that', commented Harry's mother). It was obvious Harry had a severe nose and sinus allergy (swollen, pale and blistered nose lining, dramatic 'allergy-attack' features at the highest point of his nose). He was wheezing loudly despite taking his prescribed anti-asthma therapy.

Allergy testing revealed strong positive reactions to tree and grass pollens.

His new management restored his nasal lining to normal and it was then stabilized further with a nose spray (see Chapter 4). Because Harry had both nose and sinus and lung allergic challenges he was prescribed an anti-allergy drug. For the first time in years Harry's quality of life improved. He showed a dramatic recovery in his chest as his nose and sinus problems came under control. After about four weeks his asthma medication was reduced by as much as 80 per cent.

Harry now has excellent asthma control with fewer drugs being used. And he feels much more comfortable in his 'head' now that his nose is unblocked. With a grass pollen immunotherapy strategy started, there's a good chance Harry's hay fever (and, by extension, his asthma as well) may be totally reversed.

What can we conclude from this? Harry's upper airways allergy (hay fever) was impacting on his lower airways (lungs), causing asthma. Once identified and treated, Harry's out-of-control allergic hay fever came under control, dramatically improving the boy's quality of life. And his parents weren't half pleased, too.

It is now recognized internationally that asthma is but one component of a more complex and complicated interreaction of nose/sinus problems and the lungs. It's a real shame that chest specialists don't inspect the nose and sinuses as part of their overall assessment of patients suspected of having asthma. Equally, it's quite frustrating for patients to attend ear, nose and throat (ENT) specialists who will never check their very obvious coughs and wheezes.

Conclusion

All asthma, especially in children, probably begins in the nose and sinuses and spreads to involve the lungs. Asthma as a solo lung condition probably doesn't exist, there's almost always some degree of nose and sinus involvement. Treating asthma alone without addressing the associated nose and sinus problems condemns the person concerned to unnecessary anti-asthma drugs and misses the focal point of the problem. Doctors should always inspect the nose and sinuses as part of their assessment of adults and children with asthma. They should deal properly with the associated nose and sinus issues when considering how to help their asthmatic patients.

It isn't rocket science. It's more important than rocket science. It could be you or your child suffering needlessly.

4

How doctors should treat hay fever

Got hay fever? Why don't you just take an antihistamine?
STOP! That's the wrong approach. Pharmaceutical giants may plug these products on the airwaves, doctors and chemists may prescribe them or hand them out like jelly beans, but that plan just doesn't work. It may give short-term benefit (reducing the nasal irritability that leads to sneezing and a runny nose), but it does nothing for nasal congestion. And nasal congestion is the main persisting consequence of allergic nasal challenge. If doctors don't reverse the blockage they condemn patients to a miserable summer.

Let me explain why.

Every working day in my clinic people with hay fever relate how miserable their lives are. Sometimes they are children as young as five. Since children cannot always vocalize how they feel, it's up to the parents to speak on their behalf.

'He's constantly stuffed up in the nose.'

'He's always rubbing at his eyes. If he doesn't stop he'll have the eyes rubbed out of his head.'

'He says he's getting headaches. I'm worried he might have a brain tumour.'

'He's sneezing and snorting and it's driving the rest of us mad. He doesn't know how to blow his nose.'

'I'm buying boxes of paper hankies by the dozen. His pockets are bulging with screwed-up tissues.'

'He's exhausted. Look at those dark circles round his eyes.'

Often the child is also grumpy, irritable, moody and out of sorts. Those features are usually mentioned by way of handwritten notes so the parents' concerns aren't talked about in front of the child. They wonder if this is the boy or girl's true temperament or his or her response to ill-health.

With adults the complaints are up front and loud. There's no holding back or couching the language in subtle tones.

'I feel really awful.'

'I'm miserable. I just want to curl up in a ball and go to sleep.'

'I'm not sleeping properly and my wife says I snore so loudly she can't sleep either. When I wake up in the morning my mouth feels dry because I'm breathing through it all night.'

'Help!'

With all patients, adults or children, I have a strategy to identify what the real issue is, how to explain it and then how to put things right. So pretend you're in my clinic and let me set out my stall of management.

In the clinic

First I listen carefully to the complaints, trying not to interrupt so I get a feel for the severity of the symptoms. Then I pose leading questions.

- *How blocked is your nose?* This tells me the severity of swelling of the nose lining.
- *Sneezing? How often? How aggressive are the sneezing attacks?* Now I know how irritated the nose lining must be.
- *Do you have a dull ache along the forehead and cheek bones?* An answer of 'yes' suggests sinus blockage and possible sinus inflammation.
- *How are your senses of taste and smell? Can you smell perfume but not sweaty socks?* If there's a 'yes' to this, I now know the nasal swelling is stubborn and longstanding. (For some strange reason it's unpleasant smells that go first in this situation, followed eventually by all smells, good, bad or indifferent.)
- *How is your hearing? Do your ears pop? Do voices seem muffled?* If 'yes', the nasal swelling has extended to the back of the throat and involves the Eustachian tube, the narrow channel connecting to the inner ear. If the Eustachian tube is in any way obstructed there is almost always a degree of hearing impairment.
- *Do you have excess mucus flow at the back of the throat?* If 'yes', the obstruction at the top of the nose is reversing normal mucus drainage.

- *Are you coughing or wheezing? Do you feel unusually short of breath?* If so, the hay fever has inflamed the nose and sinuses so much that in turn the lungs are irritated.
- *How about your eyes? They look red. Are they itchy? Are you digging your knuckles into the corner of the eyes to relieve that itch?* A glum nod tells me that the naso-ocular reflex is sending allergy-like impulses from nose to eyes. Depending on how severe the eye irritation is, I can decide if the extra assault of pollen grains as they come into direct contact with the eye lining explains the redness, itching and swelling.
- *Does your mouth or throat itch when you eat certain foods, especially fruit?* Now I'm uncovering any hint of 'oral-allergy syndrome', where proteins in certain foods cross-react with the airborne pollen grains.

You still haven't explained why an antihistamine is the wrong approach in hay fever.

Patience, I'm getting to that.

At this point I inspect the nasal cavity (in other words I shine a very bright light up the nose and examine all the structures that can be observed). This gives an instant impression of the problem. Then, using a flexible fibrescope (as illustrated in Figure 1.2, on page 3), I inspect the nasal lining from nose tip to throat. As the fibre-scope moves along, an exact image is captured on a LCD screen. I can then point out what's going wrong and the patient (or parent) can understand better the un-wellness he or she feels (or observes). Often the images are so dramatic that people are shocked. *Now* they grasp why they're so miserable (or why their child is so out of sorts).

I explain the connection between the symptoms and what I've spotted with the fibrescope. Using a diagram of the nose and sinuses (Figure 4.1, overleaf), I describe their function and intercon-nection, as follows.

'The lining of the nose is delicate and easily irritated. Running along the inside are three shelf-like structures called *turbinates*. These clean, filter, warm and moisten the air we breathe before it enters the lungs. But if the turbinates are attacked by pollen grains they swell. If they swell a lot they block the little tubes that drain the sinuses into the nose. Now we not only have hay fever but, potentially, allergic sinusitis as well.

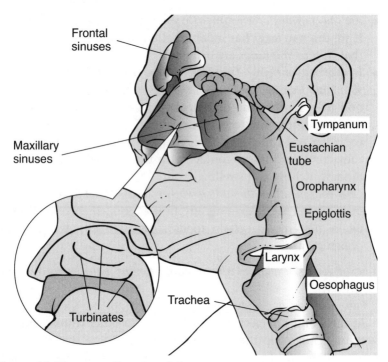

Figure 4.1 The nose, throat and sinuses

'If the swelling within the nose persists,' I continue, 'the sinuses cannot breathe, their air pockets stagnate and become a rich feeding ground for infection. The nerve link between the nose and sinuses and the lungs is agitated, causing a cough, wheezing and breathing difficulties.' I let that sink in.

'So,' I go on, 'when you say you think you have hay fever you probably think it's all a nasal problem. However, it's more complicated than that. Hay fever can involve the sinuses, eyes and lungs. It may even trigger skin irritability, in other words eczema.'

Which brings me to the point of not using antihistamines as a first-choice medicine. Antihistamines may relieve the nasal irritability (the sneezing and runny nose), but they do nothing for the blockage. And it's the blockage that causes most of the discomfort in hay fever.

'So,' I say, 'I won't use an antihistamine to help you. I'll first unblock that bunged-up nose.'

How?

'Simple,' I say. 'I'll prescribe "unblocking" drops, safe for adults and children when prescribed correctly. The only difficulty (and it's not significant) is that the drops must be used in a specific "head-back" or "head-forward" position.'

Figure 4.2 shows how these drops are administered. The patient lies on a couch or bed so that the head can bend to a 90-degree angle either forwards or backwards. *Children really only benefit from the head-back, rather than the head-forward strategy.* The idea is to allow the prescribed drops (called Betnesol, chemical name beta-methasone) to trickle around the swollen nose lining, coat all the tissue and find a resting point at the 'ceiling' level of the nose. The medicine in Betnesol slowly reduces the swelling of the nasal and turbinate linings. How long the drops are used depends on how blocked the nose is at the start of treatment. Typically the duration of the therapy can vary from five days in small children to three or even four weeks in adults.

When the nose is sufficiently unblocked, then a nose spray is used to stabilize the nasal cavity. The spray (and there are a number of excellent products) is directed into the now normal-looking

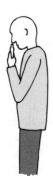

Bend head forward and hold chin in.

Hold the spray in the left hand to treat right nostril and vice versa.

If using squirts, alter the angle to wet as much as possible of the inside of the nostril.

Do not sniff too hard as this drags the solution too quickly to the back of the throat.

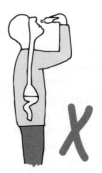

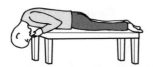

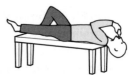

Figure 4.2 How to use nose drops and nose spray

nose in a dosage decided by your treating doctor. The purpose is to maintain the improvement that we've achieved with the Betnesol drops. If we just treat with drops and stop as soon as normality is achieved, unfortunately the nasal lining may swell again. So it's very important not only to restore the nose to health but also keep it unblocked.

The box shows a typical regime for an adult.

Betnesol nose drops: correct use

1 Get into the position suggested (see Figure 4.2, page 31).
2 Instil 2 drops into each nostril (it might be easier to have someone help you with this, as it's not easy to concentrate on the position *and* ensure you're getting the drops in properly).
3 Stay in the same position for 3 minutes.
4 After 3 minutes pinch the soft part of your nose closed. Now lift your head to its normal position (some drops may spill out at this point, but that's not important).
5 Do this twice daily (preferably morning and evening) for 14 days.
6 On day 15 start the nasal spray. (Nasacort, Flixonase, Avamys, Nasonex or Dymista are the trade names for a group of excellent nose sprays used in persisting hay fever. Dymista is a new product with the novel combination of antihistamine and a steroid medicine. As I write it's not yet on the market, so I have no personal experience of any benefit. However medical trial results that I've seen suggest it could be a winner.) The dosage is 1 squiff up into each nostril (as shown in Figure 4.2) twice daily. Continue this until review.
7 In the meantime (or at any time in the future, where this is an ongoing programme), if you get breakthrough 'head cold' symptoms, stop the spray and restart the Betnesol drops (in the same position as above) until the blockage clears. This may take as little as one to two days. Even if it takes longer, persist. The nasal spray cannot work if you are spraying it into a blocked or runny nose. The aim of this plan is to restore normal nose function.

Why do I insist on treatment with nose drops? Because by the time people (whether children or adults) contact doctors for help with hay fever their noses are usually significantly blocked. If the nasal obstruction doesn't clear with the Betnesol drops plan, I add an oral anti-allergy medicine called Singulair (chemical name montelukast) or Accolate (chemical name zafirlukast). This is especially important where there is associated coughing and wheezing. These compounds, called *leukotriene receptor antagonists*, 'mop up' one of the most important chemicals involved in nose, sinus and chest allergy.

Questions and answers: nose drops and nasal sprays

What happens afterwards?
To minimize the amount of medicine required for long-term control, I strongly recommend nasal lavage (explained in detail in Chapter 10). This involves irrigating the nasal passages with a warm water solution of salt and baking soda.

Can I still use antihistamines?
Antihistamines can be used if you're still troubled with hay fever despite the above approach (although if it's done properly that is unlikely to happen). If an antihistamine is needed, ask your doctor or pharmacist for one of the newer products. Older antihistamines caused significant drowsiness, so that people with hay fever spent most of their summers fast asleep and didn't know whether they were better or not!

Newer antihistamines include Xyzal (levocetirizine), Zirtek (cetirizine), Neoclarityn (desloratadine) and Drynol (bilastine). Older products include Piriton (chlorpheniramine maleate), Zaditen (ketotifen), Vallergan (trimeprazine tartarate) and Telfast (fexofenadine). There are a number of cheaper (called generic) variations of the above medicines so, when choosing, look for pharmaceutical name rather than commercial tag (e.g. Zirtene instead of Zirtek). Here the basic ingredient is still the same: cetirizine.

This all sounds too easy. Will it work?
Yes. Failure of treatments is usually due to the incorrect use of drops, not taking them long enough or failing to follow through with the nose spray immediately after the course of drops.

What's in Betnesol drops?
Cortisone (a steroid). This is the only medication that will successfully shrink the swollen and distorted nasal lining to normal. Provided you stick to the recommended dose you need not fear

the usual cortisone side effects. Equally, do not self-medicate with Betnesol drops without keeping your treating doctor informed. The doctor needs to know how much and how often you're taking this medication, because there is a point at which side effects might occur. (One of the many reasons I'm a big fan of nasal lavage – see Chapter 10 – is that it keeps the nasal/sinus linings clean and fresh and less likely to break down again and again. Daily nasal lavage should allow you to keep prescribed medicines to a minimum. And it's only a salt and baking soda mixture, totally harmless but very effective.)

What's in the nasal sprays?
These also contain the steroid cortisone. Again, this is the only medicine that successfully stabilizes and protects the nose and sinus linings, especially when the problem is allergy driven. (The new product Dymista contains both steroid and antihistamine medication, and could be an exciting combination for pollen-allergy sufferers.)

Steroid nasal sprays have exact doses in each 'squiff', so it's actually difficult to overdose on them. Regular use does not damage the nose, thin the nasal lining or make the lining more vulnerable to infections (or any other scare story you've heard about them). Nor does the medication get absorbed into the blood when used according to the prescriber's instructions.

Does this strategy work for all types of hay fever? Summer or all-year-round?
The kernel of dealing with all hay fever is to restore the nasal lining to normal. Failure to address that basic issue dooms the patient to unnecessary misery. But, yes, this does work both in summer-only and all-year-round hay fever.

What about the irritable eyes?
Here the safest anti-allergy eye drops contain the compound sodium cromoglycate (trade names include Opticrom, Hay-Crom and Vividrin). These are used for extra relief. Other safe products are ketotifen (trade name Zaditen), olopatadine (trade name Opatanol) and xylometalozine (trade name Otrivine-Antistin). In severe eye allergy, especially where there is swelling of the inside of the upper lids (as described in Chapter 1), steroid (cortisone) eye drops must be used for relief. However these can only be safely prescribed by

an eye specialist. He or she can monitor closely the improvement of the surface of the eye as the allergic irritation subsides and decide when to stop treatment.

Got hay fever? Why don't you just take an antihistamine?
Now you know why that's the wrong approach.

Summary

Don't take an antihistamine for relief of hay fever until you've unblocked your nose (as described in this chapter). Once that's cleared, some long-term strategy should be decided. It's not a good idea to lurch from one crisis summer to the next. It's your well-being that suffers. Remember:

- sinus problems begin as a blocked nose;
- eye irritation in hay fever also involves the nose;
- lung irritation in hay fever occurs when the nasal irritation becomes aggressive;
- a normal, healthy nose may allow you to have normal, healthy sinuses, eyes and lungs;
- stage 1 of management involves unblocking the nose with Betnesol drops as described; Stage 2 involves stabilizing the nose and sinuses with a nasal spray;
- for stubborn allergic nose problems, adding in Singulair or Accolate will often produce the final clearance.

Once we've got you better, why not consider the next stage of treatment? Here we take a long-term view on your management. Do you want to keep taking medicines throughout the summer to stay well? No? Why not consider immunotherapy, where we dramatically reduce your allergic sensitivity to pollens?

You can read about immunotherapy in the next chapter.

5

Immunotherapy as a long-term treatment for hay fever

Allergy management involves avoidance of what you are allergic to, combined with treatment of the symptoms. For example, in the nasal allergy we call hay fever, pollen-avoidance measures (as set out in Chapter 1) are advised, while the snorting and sneezing is suppressed with medication. However, while such manoeuvres and treatments are indeed very effective, they do not alter your allergic status. In other words, you are still allergic to pollen grains and will still get into trouble if the avoidance measures and treatments are relaxed or stopped. For almost everyone with an allergy this means many years (even a lifetime) of taking anti-allergy remedies.

Now a new therapy, called *immunotherapy* (which is actually a 100-year-old therapy but has recently been updated), offers the chance to significantly reduce your 'allergicness' and maybe even completely stop reactions. Immunotherapy entails taking exactly what you are allergic to, but in a modified form. At present the most convenient regime, called sublingual immunotherapy, is a soluble tablet placed under the tongue and held there for two minutes.

In North America and some European countries, immunotherapy is given by weekly injections. It's exactly the same principle, just a different mode of delivery. But this is not very patient-friendly. Taking time out to go to the same doctor, week after week, for a single injection is more than most people with an allergy are prepared to do. The under-the-tongue (sublingual) version is more acceptable as a long-term course of treatment.

In medical jargon, allergen immunotherapy blocks the allergic reaction well upstream of the inflammatory response and may even prevent nose and sinus allergy deteriorating into lung allergy (asthma). Moreover, its beneficial effect persists long after the end of the course of therapy.

Allergen immunotherapy is especially helpful with hay fever-induced nose and sinus problems. Allergen immunotherapy:

- reduces symptoms significantly;
- reduces the amount of medication needed for comfort and relief;
- reduces nose and chest sensitivity to allergic irritation;
- reduces the risk of developing other allergies.

How does it work?

Allergen immunotherapy acts by exposing you to a small amount of whatever you're allergic to. This stimulates the immune system to produce 'blocking' antibodies. In turn this reduces allergy symptoms, making you more tolerant of your allergy triggers in the future.

Grass pollen allergy symptoms are improved from the first season of treatment onwards.

Why recommend immunotherapy?

Because it's the only strategy that offers the chance to significantly reduce or even stop anti-allergy medicines. More often than not anti-allergy treatments are used daily for years, even for a lifetime. Anything safe and effective, which might ease that considerable pharmaceutical burden, is worth considering. The commitment to treatment is vital and this is important to understand, as you will be embarking on a minimum of three and possibly five years of therapy.

What are the treatments?

There are two products licensed in Britain and Ireland for grass pollen allergy sublingual immunotherapy: Grazax and Oralair. Both are soluble tablets. Ideally they are taken in the morning before breakfast. A tablet is placed under the tongue until it dissolves completely. Usually this takes no more than a minute. The remaining saliva is then swallowed. There are simple and commonsense cautions to observe, such as not taking two tablets on the same day (unless that's specifically instructed); if you miss a tablet then take one (and one only) the next day, do not double up on the missed dose. If you miss several days' treatment (maybe you left the packet at home while away), then you need to check with your treating doctor as to how to restart the programme. Too long a delay may mean the early benefits have faded. You may have to start from scratch again.

Side effects are minimal and settle to nil after a couple of weeks' continuous therapy. They include itching, tingling inside the mouth and throat, itchy ears or nausea and cramp stomach pains. These side effects tend to trouble children more than adults. In rare cases (and this has never happened in all the patients I've treated), widespread body hives (called urticaria) erupt, asthma surfaces or pre-existing asthma worsens. Severe swelling of the tongue and throat, with a general sense of feeling very unwell may also become an issue. If you (or your child) can put up with the minor discomforts, then they abate eventually (within weeks). However, severe symptoms mean immunotherapy is unwise and dangerous for you and must be stopped immediately.

Immunotherapy must be started well in advance of the pollen season to achieve the immune stimulation needed to try and induce a significant reduction in your sensitivity to grass pollen. Grazax is taken daily for 52 weeks of the year for a minimum of three years. Oralair is a six-month, pre-season medicine. Highly allergic individuals may require a five-year course for final resolution of their sensitivity.

Here I must sound a word of caution. There's nothing wrong or dangerous about immunotherapy. But there is a major issue relating to doctors knowing enough about it or how to use it (more on this in Chapter 9). If 10,000 pollen grains might fit on the point of a needle, the number of experienced allergy doctors in Britain and Ireland would fit comfortably into one single-decker bus. There aren't enough of us. Other medics such as family doctors, respiratory physicians and paediatricians know little if anything about either allergy or immunotherapy. Consequently you may experience blank stares, expressions of disinterest or cynicism, or even downright hostility, if you ask about this treatment. Ignorance is often disguised by hostility towards or dismissal of allergy in general and immunotherapy in particular.

So choose your treating doctor carefully if you wish to explore immunotherapy as a logical alternative to an all-medicines approach. If you use the internet be wary of bogus allergy clinics (there are many) and check closely on the qualifications and experience of those offering their services. For example, I am a member of the British Society for Allergy and Clinical Immunology (BSACI) and the European Academy of Allergy and Clinical Immunology (EAACI). Is the doctor you're thinking of visiting involved in either or both of those societies? If not, why not? Maybe this person is not a qualified doctor. Check and double check. It's your health (and money, for these are private clinics) that's at risk.

A short, sharp way to make hay fever go away

Finally, there is another product called Kenalog that is occasionally used to treat hay fever. Kenalog (chemical name triamcinolone) is a long-acting steroid (cortisone) injection. It comes as a single ampoule shot and lasts approximately 6 weeks at its 40 milligrams strength.

Most specialists in allergy and ENT disorders avoid Kenalog because of potential side effects. The drug is a steroid and consequently has the potential to cause a number of problems, including suppression of natural cortisone production, dimpling of the skin and fatty tissue underneath the injection site, thinning of bones and wasting of muscle and tendons. So why even consider it?

Well, there is a sub-group of severe hay fever sufferers for whom standard treatments cannot work. This includes those with significant mental or physical disabilities who cannot manage the daily ritual of anti-hay fever therapies. Also, long-distance lorry drivers and machine workers need to be alert all the time. If the grogginess of hay fever combined with the side effects of antihistamines impairs their concentration, a serious accident could happen.

A single, once-a-season, once-a-year injection of Kenalog will not cause side effects. Indeed it offers hay fever sufferers a decent quality of life during a time of year when we all like to be outdoors. It MUST NOT, however, be used more than once a year.

I use it quite a lot for a select group of patients (such as those mentioned). I also give Kenalog to anyone with severe hay fever doing important exams, getting married, etc. This is when I feel there must be total hay fever control so that big life events can be faced with confidence. For example, studies show that students with hay fever lose as much as 15 per cent of performance during major exams.

Equally I don't want a beautiful bride to walk up the aisle on her big day snorting and sniffing, tears streaming down her mascara-streaked face. It could give the groom the wrong impression. *Does she love me or not? Is it last-minute nerves or a change of heart?* To make sure everyone looks good and says the right thing at the crucial point, I give Kenalog about ten days before the wedding. That way the bride can say 'I do' with confidence and not 'I, I, I, I – *Aaaaaccchhhooo!* Oh, I feel miserable. What were you asking there?'

The celebrant doesn't want to stand with his face covered in sneeze droplets and have to pretend he's not in the least bit bothered. And the groom shouldn't be having second thoughts at that critical moment. Do I really want to marry this car-crash of an allergic wreck?

A shot of Kenalog has prevented a lot of examination disasters and allowed many brides to look beautiful on their special day. What happens after that is out of my control.

6

Allergy testing in hay fever

How do you find out what type of pollen is causing your hay fever? And what can be done about it?

Your doctor has inspected your nose and decided that your problem is almost certainly hay fever. To decide a long-term strategy, the doctor will want to know exactly what you're allergic to (and so do you), so will order an allergy test. I don't want to confuse you with science or medical jargon, but let's now explore the basics of allergy.

What is allergy?

An allergy occurs when the body's immune system overreacts to normally harmless substances (called allergens). These substances may be in the air or may be things you touch or eat. So the term allergen means anything that triggers an allergic reaction.

If you are an allergic person, and you come into contact with an allergen, your immune system produces a certain type of antibody (called *IgE*). Other cells release chemicals such as histamine that cause the symptoms you experience (blocked nose, itchy eyes, sneezing, etc.).

Common allergens

This book deals with hay fever, so I'm going to focus on the allergens that cause nasal symptoms: almost always grass, tree, weed and shrub pollens. About 15 to 18 per cent of the population are exquisitely sensitive (allergic) to pollen grains. As pollen enters the nose it triggers sneezing and a runny nose, followed soon after by swelling of the delicate nasal lining. Very soon the nose becomes blocked. If the nasal blockage persists, the natural openings into the sinuses (from the inside of the nose) are obstructed. Now the soft lining of the sinuses become irritated and sinus symptoms such as facial pain, pressure and headaches along the front of the forehead erupt.

Allergy symptoms

These depend on which part of the body is affected. For example, hay fever affects the eyes and nose, causing sneezing, a runny or stuffy, blocked nose, watery and itchy eyes, and an irritated and itchy throat.

Eczema (also called dermatitis) is an allergic affliction of the skin causing itchy, red rashes.

Asthma is an allergic challenge to the respiratory system causing wheezing, breathlessness, chest tightness and a cough.

Allergies to foods, bites or stings can cause hives (doctors prefer the term urticaria, because it's a strange term and using out of the ordinary words makes us feel important).

Diagnosing allergy

There are three types of allergy test.

1 RAST (radioallergosorbent test). This identifies exactly what you are allergic to through a blood sample. There are practical difficulties with RAST testing: it is expensive, the results take weeks to return and there is a limit to the number of substances that can be tested.
2 Serum IgE, another blood test, checks the number of allergy cells circulating in your body. This tells you how allergic you are but *not* what you're allergic to.
3 Skin-prick allergy testing. This is the commonest procedure used in allergy clinics, and I'll now explain it in detail.

The surface of the skin is rich in mast cells. To cut through a lot of unnecessary medical jargon, mast cells hold the body's memory for allergy, in other words the cells recognize what you are allergic to.

There are mast cells on the surface of the eyes, nose and sinuses, mouth and tongue, and throughout your breathing and eating tracts. They also run along the surface of the gut. In allergic reactions the mast cells 'explode', releasing a number of chemicals that cause problems. Where the reaction is localized (e.g. in pollen hay fever, they are confined to the nose, sinuses and eyes) the problems stay localized (itchy eyes, sneezing, blocked nose, sinus congestion). Where the reaction is widespread (e.g. if someone highly allergic is exposed to shellfish) the mast cell eruption can be so aggressive that it causes a total body (and occasionally fatal) response.

With a skin-prick allergy test the doctor places a concentrated drop of allergy extract onto the skin (usually the forearm but occasionally the back, especially in small children). Each drop contains an individual test substance such as dust mite, cat hair, horsehair, grass pollen or a particular food. Not every food is available in test form and occasionally fresh food will be used.

The test drop is brought into direct contact with the skin mast cells by pricking the surface with a sterile needle point and allowing the fluid to seep to a lower level. If you are allergic to a specific substance the mast cells underneath will 'explode' and a reaction (called a 'wheal and flare') appears. Simply put, the wheal is a red, itchy blister that forms over the test extract and the flare is the associated redness of the skin.

The presence of the central blister confirms to the doctor that you are allergic to the substance administered, while the intensity of any surrounding skin redness indicates how strongly allergic you are. Small reactions are not as important as large swellings, while large and very irregular reactions suggest a person is highly allergic to a substance. Large and very irregular reactions to food extracts suggest the possibility of a very aggressive and total body allergic response if that food is consumed. The final interpretation depends on what symptoms you have, what the doctor discovers when he examines you and what reactions show on testing. It's easy to perform an allergy test: the skill lies in interpreting the result and linking it to the patient's symptoms.

Questions and answers: allergy testing

Why is allergy testing important?
Finding out what you are allergic to is an important first step to effective allergy treatment. When combined with a detailed

medical history, allergy testing can identify the specific pollens that trigger your hay fever.

Who can be tested for allergies?
Adults and children of any age can be tested for allergies.

How are skin-prick tests interpreted?
A positive result is measured in millimetres of central wheal and outer flare (flare here meaning the redness of the skin). There are positive (histamine) and negative (saline) controls to compare against and thus ensure the accuracy of the result.

With foods, a wheal of 6 mm and greater suggests that particular food will trigger an allergic reaction. The greater the size of the wheal, the more likely that the reaction will be aggressive.

With environmental allergens (such as dust mites, pollens and animal hair), the size of the wheal and flare is important but does not always reflect the symptoms. For example a patient will occasionally show a very large wheal and flare (say to dust mites) but not show many symptoms. Equally a relatively small reaction (say to cat hair in someone only recently exposed to cats) is usually very important, as within a year of continuous exposure the allergic reaction will probably have increased significantly (as will the patient's symptoms).

How long does it take to get skin test results?
Skin testing is fast and positive reactions usually appear within 20 minutes. Sometimes redness and swelling can occur several hours after skin testing. The delayed reaction usually disappears in 24 to 48 hours, but should be reported to the allergy doctor or nurse.

Is skin testing painful?
Skin tests cause little or no pain. However, positive reactions cause annoying itchy red bumps that look and feel like mosquito bites. The itching and bumps are gone usually within 30 minutes.

Do any medicines interfere with allergy skin tests?
Yes. Antihistamines and specific antidepressants block the 'wheal and flare' response of skin-prick tests. Before attending for an allergy test you must not take tablets or liquid antihistamine medicines (these are found in most cough medicines). Antihistamine and steroid creams are also potentially troublesome for the same

reason. Ideally you should not take steroid tablets, but this is not vital and will not significantly interfere with the result. If you have any doubt about medications please check with your treating allergist.

When are blood allergy tests used?
Blood allergy test are used if:

- you are taking a medicine that interferes with skin testing and cannot stop taking it;
- you suffer from a skin condition so severe that there is no normal skin on which to perform the test;
- testing with a strong allergen might cause an especially unpleasant positive reaction.

How long does it take to get blood test results?
Because the blood sample must be sent to a laboratory for testing, it takes many days, even weeks, to get results.

If something significant shows on testing, what anti-allergy advice am I likely to be offered?

- Environmental control based on allergy test results that confirm your hay fever is caused by airborne allergens such as grass pollen. There's more on this overleaf.
- Immunotherapy (explained in Chapter 5).

The bottom line on allergy testing is this: the result must be interpreted in combination with your symptoms (your sense of un-wellness), what the doctor finds when examining your nose and the outcome of other tests. When the doctor has the whole package, he or she can then conclude with some certainty that your positive skin allergy test truly reflects the cause of your hay fever. That decided, she then offers appropriate anti-allergy advice. The more experienced the doctor, the wiser the advice you'll be offered.

What about changing the environment around me to reduce exposure to allergy triggers?

Yes, you can do that. I would recommend you to follow the self-help tips I gave you in Chapter 1 and to follow the dietary advice given there and in Chapter 11.

Should I move to another country?

No, for the reasons I explained in Chapter 1. Basically you carry your 'allergicness' with you wherever you go. While you may feel better in the short term because of being separated from your allergic triggers, in time you become sensitized to and react to the new locality. Sorry, I'd like to offer you more comfort, but that's the hard reality of allergy.

Environmental control of dust mite and animal hair allergy

If allergy testing shows you are allergic to indoor allergens such as dust mites and pets, then the following manoeuvres are certainly worthwhile.

Dust mites, pollens, moulds and pet hair are the most important cause of sinusitis. Because they may not always be easily avoided, try minimizing the 'allergy load' in your home as described below. At the end there are some practical tips on pollen-allergy avoidance strategies.

Dust mites live comfortably in mattresses, pillows, duvets, blankets, carpets, soft furnishings, curtains and similar fabrics. Female mites lay up to 50 eggs at a time, with a new generation produced every three weeks. Each mite produces about 20 waste particles every day. When working on anti-dust mite regimes, concentrate on the bedroom.

- If your bedding (mattress, pillows, eiderdowns, bolsters) contains wool, kapok, cotton, horsehair, feathers or down with synthetic materials, change to polyester or Dacron.
- Buy blankets and curtains made of synthetic fibres.
- Get rid of down, winceyette and flannel materials.
- Get rid of carpets and rugs. Here there really should be no compromise. Mites also thrive in carpeting, no matter how tight the pile. People with mite allergy should have wooden (no unsealed cracks), linoleum, cork-tiled or parquet floors. These surfaces are so much easier to clean and run a wet mop over.
- Get rid of cushions not filled with synthetic materials, as well as anything made from wool or cotton.
- Minimize dust collectors such as heavy curtains, bookshelves, tapestries, etc.
- Paint rather than wallpaper the walls of the bedroom.

- Get rid of teddy bears and other soft toys. Special 'life-is-not-worth-living-without' soft toys should be washed at least once a week and each morning put into the deep freeze for about three hours to kill off mites.
- Open the bedroom windows for at least three hours every day, even in very cold weather.
- Use a damp cloth when dusting. Anything else only redistributes the dust.
- Choose lightweight curtains that are quick and easy to wash at temperatures around 58° C. Consider roller blinds.
- Remove fabric-covered headboards.
- Use only a vacuum cleaner with a pollen-and-dust filtration unit. Vacuum and damp dust at least once a week.
- A bed with a plain wooden or metal base is preferable to a divan.
- Where bunk beds are in use, the person with sinus problems should sleep in the top bunk.
- Do not allow pets into the bedroom of a person with sinus problems.
- Do not smoke, or allow anyone else to smoke, in the presence of someone with sinus problems or in any other room that person is likely to use.
- Don't have the radiator on much in the bedroom, perhaps just enough to take the chill out of the air. Mites love warm temperatures.
- All clothes, shoes and socks should be put away in drawers and not left lying around the room. Don't hang clothes on hooks on the backs of doors.
- If possible, have built-in wardrobes rather than free-standing units.
- Mattresses, pillows and duvets should be aired regularly. If there is a spell of good weather, get the bedding outside and into the air and beat the mattress to clear excess dust.
- Encase the mattress, pillows and duvet with a protective cover that is comfortable to lie on, but does not permit dust mites to penetrate. There are a number of companies dealing with these products and the price differences between them are very significant.
- Choose your vacuum cleaner carefully. The best machines (and

unfortunately the most expensive) are those with very efficient dust filtration units. This means the collected dust is retained and not recirculated. Look for models produced by Medivac, Electrolux, Miele and Dyson. Make sure the supplier hasn't removed the filtration bag (it does happen).

- When you are vacuuming and damp dusting, try to do a thorough job at least once a week and remember to go under the bed with the vacuum cleaner.

NB: If you have sinus problems and smoke cigarettes don't waste time, money and effort on anti-allergy manoeuvres. If you continue to smoke you undo the good that the above measures might achieve. Even more important, if your child is troubled with his or her nose and sinuses and you, your husband, wife, granny, uncle, babyminder or whoever, smokes such that your child passively inhales, then again don't bother with anti-allergy programmes. Cigarette smoking makes all allergy problems worse.

7

Hay fever and allergic irritability in children

Hay fever makes people feel quite miserable. About that, there is no argument. However, hay fever in children, if unrecognized (maybe it's been misdiagnosed as a summer head cold) or badly managed, can take a significant toll on emotional as well as physical well-being.

For years I've been dealing with children troubled by multiple allergy problems and wondered how they get through a full school day. What with their itchy eczematous skin, their snuffly and irritable noses and wheezy chests, they carry a significant burden of ill-health. Adults know how to complain (and rarely hold back), whereas some children don't know any better. They think everyone goes around with a bunged-up nose, wheezy chest and almost perpetual tiredness. If the hay fever is especially troublesome, the child may experience intermittent hearing loss. One day she's bright and alert in class, interreacting and cooperating. Next day she seems distant and detached, ignoring questions or not fully grasping what's going on. The teachers are at a loss to explain these variations in attentiveness and the girl's parents can't quite understand the situation either. It's not uncommon for these children to be labelled 'difficult'.

Hay fever also provokes intense fatigue. If affected children are not treated they miss out on ordinary children's activities and can be isolated and ignored. They're not picked for the football team even though they love the game. And if they're picked they're usually last choice and then put in goal, out of harm's way. Secretly they'd love to be strikers, fast footed and skilful. They know they're well able to take the ball around defences. If only they could get the chance. If only they didn't feel so tired all the time. If only they didn't have to stop every five yards to blow their noses, if only they didn't have to take a puff of their asthma inhalers in front of everyone. If only, if only . . .

Persisting nasal allergy such as occurs in hay fever can often trigger dramatic problems for children. With allergy on the rise worldwide (more on this in Chapter 9), the plight of the untreated allergic child is not a happy one.

I've been talking about this for years, to the point of being considered a crank. Then an article (H. P. van Bever and P. C. Potter, 'Making the allergic child happy: Treating more than symptoms', *Clinical and Experimental Allergy Reviews* 6, Feb 2006, 6–9) appeared in a reputable medical journal and summarized my observations to a tee. Suddenly I knew how right I'd been. Now I realized that I wasn't the only one making these comments. The difference was that while my observations were no more than just that, observations, the authors of this piece had the scientific background to support their claims.

The term *allergic irritability syndrome* has been coined to explain the many unpleasant symptoms and features children with untreated allergic rhino-sinusitis (ARS) may show. Allergic rhino-sinusitis is a fancy medical term for allergy-driven nose and sinus problems.

Effects of allergic rhino-sinusitis

Here goes. Children with unrecognized ARS (as can occur with hay fever) have:

- a significantly impaired quality of life;
- significant learning difficulties;
- a lower ability to achieve different types of knowledge (factual, conceptual and application) compared with healthy children;
- nasal blockage and irritation (sneezing, rubbing at the nose to relieve the itch);
- dark circles around the eyes with puffiness of the lower lids;
- poor concentration, disruptive behaviour and unexplained mood swings.

They may also suffer sleep apnoea (see Chapter 8), snoring and disturbed sleep patterns. This in turn leads to daytime drowsiness, grumpy mood and poor school performance. In severe cases ARS may cause or at least contribute to attention deficit hyperactivity disorder (ADHD). If fluid collects in the inner ear (medical term:

serous otitis media), this may cause impaired hearing. They may suffer repeated 'head colds' that go down to the chest (which is really an untreated nose and sinus allergy triggering early asthma).

I recall one six-year-old boy who told his parents that he felt angry all the time when unwell with his allergic sinusitis. This is sad and unnecessary, as nasal allergy is easily managed, especially in children. The treatment strategies outlined in Chapter 4 apply to children as well as adults.

Let's now look at the common effects of persisting hay fever in children.

Nasal congestion

Hay fever is a common cause of chronic (long-lasting and ongoing) nasal congestion in children. Sometimes a child's nose is congested (obstructed) to the point that he or she breathes through the mouth, especially while sleeping.

If the congestion is left untreated this forces air currents through the mouth. The strength of the air changes the way the soft bones of the face grow. The features may become abnormally elongated, causing the teeth to come in at an improper angle as well as creating an overbite. Braces or other dental treatments may be necessary to correct these problems.

Ear infections

Hay fever can lead to inflammation in the ear and may cause fluid accumulation, which in turn can trigger ear infections and impaired hearing. If this happens when the child is learning to talk, poor speech development may result. Hay fever can also cause earaches and ear itching, popping and fullness ('stuffed-up ears').

Allergic diseases and cognitive impairment

Sneezing, wheezing, watery eyes and a runny nose aren't the only symptoms of allergic diseases. Many people with nasal allergy also report feeling 'slower' and drowsy. When their allergies act up they have trouble concentrating and remembering. This can be a particular problem for children in school.

For instance, nasal allergy can be associated with:

- decreased ability to concentrate and function;
- activity limitation;
- decreased decision-making capacity;
- impaired hand–eye coordination;
- impaired memory;
- irritability;
- sleep disorders;
- fatigue;
- missed days at work or school;
- school injuries.

Causes

Experts believe the main factors contributing to cognitive impairment of people with nasal allergies are sleep interruptions and over-the-counter (OTC) medications.

Secondary factors, such as blockage of the Eustachian tube, can also cause hearing problems that impair learning and comprehension. Constant nose blowing and coughing can interrupt concentration and the learning process, and allergy-related absences can cause children to miss school and subsequently fall behind.

Sleep disruption

Chronic nasal congestion can cause difficulty in breathing, especially at night. If your child has a significant nasal allergy he or she may awaken a dozen times a night. Falling asleep again can be difficult, cutting short the total number of sleep hours. Losing just a few hours of sleep can lead to a significant decrease in your child's ability to function. Prolonged loss of sleep can cause difficulty in concentration, inability to remember things and can contribute to accidents. Night after night of interrupted sleep can cause serious decreases in learning ability and performance in school.

Over-the-counter medications

Many over-the-counter sinus therapies (especially antihistamines) adversely affect mental functioning. Indeed, some allergy therapies may even cause cognitive or mental impairment, such as drowsiness, blurred vision or slower than usual decision-making.

Problems at school

An early pollen season may trigger troublesome hay fever during the school year. For some children this means absences due to allergy flare-ups. Here are some of the problems to look out for so that the condition can be properly diagnosed and treated, as well as some suggestions for helping the child who has an allergy.

- *Dust irritation*: reducing dust in the home will be helpful to most allergic family members. At school, children with allergy problems should sit away from any blackboards to prevent irritation from chalk dust.

- *School pets*: furry animals in school may cause problems for children who have an allergy. If your child's problems are worse at school, it could be the class pet.

- *Allergy problems and physical education*: sports are a big part of the school day. Having hay fever, or other allergy-related conditions such as asthma, does not mean eliminating these activities. Often medication administered by using an inhaler is prescribed before exercise to control the symptoms. Children with asthma and other allergic diseases should be able to participate in any sport the child chooses – provided the doctor's advice is followed.

- *Dry air*: with the onset of cold weather, using a humidifier to accompany forced air heating systems may be helpful in some regions of the country. Adding a small amount of moisture to dry air makes breathing easier for most people. However, care should be taken not to allow the humidity above 40 per cent, which promotes the growth of dust mites and mould.

- *Changes in behaviour*: children cannot always vocalize their annoying or painful symptoms. Their discomfort may manifest as behaviour problems. Be on the alert for possible allergies if your child has bouts of irritability, temper tantrums or decreased ability to concentrate in school. These may be signs of allergic irritability syndrome. Sometimes allergic children are badly behaved and have short attention spans. Needless to say their schoolwork suffers. When children's allergies are properly treated, their symptoms, behaviour and school performance can improve dramatically.

Jack

Jack, aged eight, is a problem child at home and at school. He seems constantly agitated, ill at ease with himself and disruptive. His teachers complain that he's troublesome, irritable, cranky and hard to handle. When they mention this to his parents they hear their own concerns echoed by Jack's mum and dad. They too find the boy difficult.

In case there's a physical cause for his behaviour, Jack is brought to the family doctor for a check-up. Within the first few minutes of the consultation the doctor notices how much Jack is agitated by his nose. He's constantly rubbing at it, dragging his sleeve along the nostril openings, snorting and snuffling. When the doctor inspects the inside lining of Jack's nose he realizes immediately that the boy has an aggressive nasal allergy. He arranges a battery of tests, including an allergy screen. Surprisingly the only abnormal reaction to show up is that Jack has a strong horsehair allergy. 'That makes no sense,' complain both parents. 'We're miles away from any horses and Jack doesn't even like going near them.' But the family doctor, wise man that he is, recognizes that something has to be irritating Jack's nose and sinuses. He advises the boy's parents to check their house carefully for horse-hair.

Two days later he gets a delighted telephone call. Jack sleeps in a room on his own. But there is a spare bed in that room for the occasional visitor. The bed was inherited from an elderly uncle and the mattress is stuffed with horsehair. Jack uses the bed as a trampoline. Every time he jumps up and down on it he disturbs the horsehair, which enters his nose and sinuses, in turn causing havoc with their delicate membranes. This is the background allergic challenge to Jack's health.

Out go the horsehair bed and mattress. Jack's room is steam cleaned to remove any residual traces of horsehair. Then Jack's troublesome nasal allergy is successfully treated with medicine.

The boy improves dramatically. His mood, personality, temperament and behaviour recover to normal limits within a week. Jack's parents are astonished. Jack's teachers are delighted. Jack's doctor is pleased as Punch at his diagnostic skills. And Jack is a much more contented child. Jack has been suffering from allergic irritability syndrome.

Jack is fortunate. However, not every doctor has the insight to check for this condition and the skill to know how to manage it correctly. There are a lot of unhappy Jacks in the world who don't know what it's like to have a normal, functioning and not-irritated nose. And there are many Jacks with hay fever being treated for summer 'head colds' and who suffer misery each year because of this ignorance. That said, with correct management doctors can turn unhappy Jacks into normal, lively children. It's easy to do and so rewarding to the treating doctor, the child and his or her parents.

8

How hay fever causes sleep apnoea and hives

Simple medical problems can surface in strange ways.

In the USA police confronted the parents of a seven-year-old boy and questioned them about physical abuse. The next-door neighbour reported that the child was regularly awake during the night, screaming in a state of terror. The parents admitted this but couldn't explain the situation. They denied abuse, physical or otherwise. A local doctor checked the boy and found no sign of abuse but significant breathing problems. He couldn't breathe through his nose and his chin was dropped in a reflexive, self-protective manner. The parents claimed he had been like that since infancy but didn't think it unusual.

The boy was admitted to hospital and discovered to have severe sleep apnoea – intermittent and recurring episodes where he stopped breathing. Examined under anaesthetic he had adenoid swelling so large it obstructed his nose completely (the adenoid is spongy tissue located at the back of the throat that can block nose breathing). Surgical removal produced a dramatic and instant cure. The seven-year-old started to sleep normally and there were no more night terrors. The neighbour was thanked. The police backed off. Order was restored.

Sleep apnoea

The case described above shows how a blocked or obstructed nose, whether due to hay fever or not, can cause a multitude of medical problems, some simple and others more problematic. In adults and children the usual cause is an allergic swelling of the nasal lining, often due to a grass pollen allergy – in other words, hay fever. Children can also get a blockage at the back of the throat due to enlarged adenoids. Interference with sleep can become a major issue here. The term *sleep apnoea* has been coined to identify this collection of symptoms.

In plain English this means the nose is so obstructed that the adult or child cannot breathe through it properly at night. The person snores heavily and the pattern of snoring is something like this: snore, snore, snore, snore, snore, snore, *snooooorrrreeee, snoooooorrrrrreeeeee, snoooooooorrrrreeeeee* . . . no breathing at all . . . for quite some time . . . *SNORRRRRRRRTTTTTTT*, yawn, more normal breathing and then back to snore, snore, snore, etc. The no-breathing episodes can last for 20, 30 or even 40 seconds at a time and this pattern continues through the night. The end result is recurring spells without oxygen that deprive the snorer (and anyone unfortunate enough to be in the same room) of restful, restorative sleep.

While this might read as amusing, in reality it's a serious health concern. For adults, persisting sleep apnoea can put pressure on the cardiovascular system. More common effects include:

- excessive daytime sleepiness, e.g. falling asleep at work, while driving, during conversation or when watching TV;
- irritability, short temper;
- morning headaches;
- forgetfulness;
- changes in mood or behaviour;
- anxiety or depression;
- decreased interest in sex.

In children it leads to daytime drowsiness, grumpy mood and poor school performance. In severe cases it may cause or at least contribute to ADHD.

It is estimated that the proportion of children with blocked noses, be it due to allergy or swollen adenoids or tonsils, could be as high as 25 per cent. That's a lot of kids with disturbed sleep (among other symptoms). And it means there are a lot of parents out there wondering just what *is* wrong with their child.

Persisting hay fever, or all-year-round hay fever (as described in Chapter 2), can leave the person concerned with a seriously blocked nose. When the obstruction reaches a critical point, usually when as little as 60 per cent of the nasal airway is obstructed, sleep apnoea becomes a problem. For children as well as adults. Don't ignore it. Sleep apnoea is a major quality of life issue and can be dangerous if not addressed.

Hives

If this section seems repetitive then I apologize. However there's no other way to explain the link between hay fever and hives, or urticaria, than by going back over some of the material I dealt with in Chapters 2 and 4 – and have another look at Figure 4.1, on page 30, showing the nose, throat and sinuses.

The lining of the nose is delicate and easily damaged. Running along the inside are three shelf-like structures called turbinates, which clean, filter, warm and moisten the air we breathe before it enters the lungs. But the turbinates are easily injured. Ignoring physical trauma, any challenge that aggressively irritates the nasal lining may cause the turbinates to swell. The challenge can range from infection to allergy, from cigarette smoking to inhaling chemical vapours, etc. When the turbinates swell they block the little tubes that drain the sinuses into the nose. Now we not only have a nose problem but the beginning of sinusitis. If the swelling within the nose persists the sinuses cannot breathe, their air pockets stagnate and become a rich feeding ground for infection. Running along the ceiling of the nose is an exquisitely delicate nerve ending that transmits the sensations of taste and smell to the brain. With prolonged pressure on this nerve from turbinate swelling these sensations fade.

The first to go is the sense of smell, usually a subtle and gradual loss over some months. Once the sense of smell has almost totally disappeared, the sense of taste becomes impaired. And it is the sense of taste for spice that wilts at the beginning. Now the person with hay fever finds most foods taste bland and goes for spicier products. Unwittingly, he or she consumes higher amounts of the additives used by the food industry to spice up its products. Chief culprit in this group is monosodium glutamate (MSG for short), also known as E621, a widely used flavouring agent in pre-packed, prepared and takeaway foods, especially Chinese, Indian, Thai and similar Oriental cuisine.

Jo

Jo is a 19-year-old student. She did exceptionally well in her final state examinations and now studies law in Dublin. Jo also has recurring hay fever with impaired senses of smell and taste. Jo grew up in a small county on the south coast of Ireland. Before moving to university she lived at home with her parents and had a healthy diet with mainly home-cooked food. But everything home-cooked tasted rather bland and Jo kept asking for something with a bit of spice in it. Mother refused. She preferred good, wholesome produce. She rarely used tins, packets, bottles or artificial stock cubes when preparing dinner. So Jo's wish for spice went unsatisfied.

Once Jo left to continue her studies she started to lead her own life, away from the constraints of her parents. She preferred the city night lights to the college library. She wanted experiences far removed from small-town Ireland. And she didn't want to waste time cooking. So she ate out a lot, or bought in, or grabbed fast and easy foods such as cup-a-soups, instant rice dishes, instant curries and pre-cooked spicy chicken wings. The easier the food was to prepare, the more attractive it was to Jo. And she enjoyed this produce better; she could actually taste something for a change. It at least had a tang to revitalize her jaded palate.

Unwittingly, Jo was swallowing a significant number of food additives. The tang in her diet was created by chemicals, mainly monosodium glutamate.

One evening she came out in a very itchy rash, which she recognized as hives. The rash subsided with an antihistamine. Then another time her upper lips swelled. The hives returned with a vengeance and it took days and a lot of antihistamines to calm her skin. Finally, one evening after a Chinese meal, Jo's lips, face and tongue swelled. Her sinuses became inflamed, painful and congested. The hives returned and this time didn't go away, despite double the usual dosage of antihistamines.

An ingredient in the Chinese meal was peanuts, and Jo concluded she had become allergic to peanuts. This frightened her because she knew that some people can get life-threatening reactions if they have a strong allergy to peanuts. So she went to an allergy centre to find out what was happening.

Allergy testing showed Jo had a strong grass pollen allergy. This was causing her nasal obstruction but certainly not her hives and facial swellings. None of the foods tested provoked a positive response. Conclusion: Jo's allergic reactions were not due to a food allergy. 'So what then,' asked Jo, 'could be causing this?' Fibre-optic inspection of her nasal cavity showed a grossly swollen nasal lining with fluid 'blistering' along the upper turbinates. More importantly, the swelling was interfering with the delicate nerve ending carrying the sensations of taste and smell to Jo's brain.

It was explained that to get better she had to avoid specific E numbers (the chemical additives put in certain food products to colour, flavour and preserve). She would also start a treatment plan to restore her nasal lining to normal and recover her lost senses of taste and smell. With full recovery she would enjoy good, wholesome food and not be so inclined to go for spice in her diet. Jo was also informed that if she followed this plan she would improve very quickly.

So what should people with hay fever eat?

Adults and children with hay fever (especially those in the 'all-year-round' category described in Chapter 2) look for tangier, spicier foods and flavourings. Unfortunately almost all tang and spice is artificially created using chemicals. People with hay fever can unwittingly make their condition worse (and add in an extra problem) by using artificially flavoured ingredients, especially in Indian and Chinese dishes.

The food and drink industry uses many chemical additives and by law the manufacturer must inform the consumer what compounds are in the can or tin or packet. Nowadays each additive is labelled by number and with the letter E attached (known as 'E numbers'). As part of Jo's overall management she had to avoid the following food additives (E number and original chemical name included):

E122 (tartrazine)
E104 (quinoline yellow)
E107 (yellow 2g)
E110 (sunset yellow)
E122 (azorubine)
E123 (amaranth)
E124 (ponceau 4R)
E127 (erythrosine)
E128 (red 2g)
E131 (patent blue)
E132 (indigo carmine)
E120–E219 inclusive (the benzoates)
E621, E622 and E623 (the glutamates)

Especially she had to look out for E621, monosodium glutamate, a widely used flavouring in snack foods, savouries, gravy mixes, stock cubes, and packet and tinned soups, as well as in Indian, Chinese and other Oriental foods.

Jo was told to avoid any product where there was poor labelling or where the label said 'contains permitted additives', 'contains permitted colourings and flavourings' or 'colourings and flavourings'. Products coloured red, orange, yellow, blue, lemon or green were banned as they might contain one of the listed agents. If she was unsure about the safety of any product, she was told not to buy it.

Jo was also warned that – for reasons not fully understood – once withdrawn, the casual reintroduction of the banned additives could trigger very aggressive reactions. Dubbed 'heightened hypersensitivity', it's as if the body is taking a breather from all the junk thrown at it. The next time one of the banned chemicals enters the system it will explode with allergic activity, producing hives, facial swelling, tongue swelling and even narrowing of the throat.

Jo managed to stick to her new regime. With her nasal allergy successfully treated Jo improved dramatically. She's still sticking to the additive-free diet and remains well to this day. She still longs for the occasional Chinese takeaway.

There's no pleasing some people.

9

Why hay fever has reached
epidemic proportions

The number of people, especially children, troubled with hay fever has increased over the last decade. Experts in immunology and allergy have calculated that more than one in four UK and Irish citizens experiences hay fever – compared with one in eight in the early 1980s. Fifty per cent of this group are allergic to grass pollen.

The statistics from the USA are even more startling. There hay fever affects 25 per cent of the population, with between 10 and 30 per cent of adults and 40 per cent of children suffering nasal allergy. Over $1 billion is spent treating the condition and many school and workplace days are lost due to the effects of hay fever. It's considered that these figures may be an underestimate, as the allergy symptoms are often mistaken as 'head colds'.

This increase in hay fever reflects the surge in all allergy-related conditions. For example asthma is increasing at a phenomenal rate. A relatively uncommon ailment in the 1970s, it now affects more than a quarter of UK and Irish citizens. This surge is also putting an extra burden on already overstretched health services. Unfortunately in the UK and Ireland there aren't enough facilities to deal with the demand for allergy investigation. In the UK this was investigated by a House of Commons committee and its findings make for depressing reading. In short the committee found a 'serious epidemic' of allergy and the Department of Health agreed. Allergy care in the NHS was totally inadequate at all levels with a postcode lottery of premium care. In Ireland it's no better; indeed it may be even worse.

The following statistics highlight the problem.

- Eighteen million people in the UK (out of a population of over 60 million) have some type of allergy.

- Three million will need to see a specialist in allergies because of multi-organ involvement (in other words allergy affecting more than one area: eyes, nose, chest, skin, etc.) or because of the complexity of the condition.
- Children are particularly affected. Over 40,000 of the children born each year will develop an allergy or allergies.
- One child in 50 has a nut allergy, apart from other food allergies.
- Allergy has become more complex and severe. At least 10 per cent of children and young adults with allergy have more than one allergic disorder.
- The NHS has six full-time specialist allergy centres – and fewer than 30 consultant allergy doctors. Many of these doctors are employed in research and so their time for clinical work (in other words dealing with people who have allergies) is restricted. Some parts of the country have no specialist allergists and family doctors in these areas have no one to turn to for practical advice.

Difficulties in getting a diagnosis

So what happens to those with allergies when they need specialist help? Quite often it turns out to be a frustrating experience. Consider this typical runaround of a boy with troublesome atopic (allergic) eczema. His main problem is his skin and that's what motivates his parents to seek expert attention. While they are with the dermatologist (skin doctor) they might mention that the boy is 'chesty' (that's his asthma). 'That's not my area,' they're told, 'you must take him to a chest doctor.' At the chest doctor's, they wonder about the boy's constant blocked nose and repeated 'head colds' (hay fever). 'That's not my problem,' trumpets the chest doctor, 'you must take him to an ear, nose and throat doctor.' At the ENT doctor's, they mention that the boy rubs at his eyes a lot and the whites are very red (conjunctivitis). 'Take him to an eye doctor,' they are advised.

Why an ENT doctor won't look at the eyes as part of his investigation of the nasal problem escapes logic. Why the chest physician refuses to inspect the nasal cavity when assessing the possible asthma symptoms is equally illogical.

This referral from one department to another is disillusioning for children and parents. It suggests a lack of understanding of the background problem. Could this boy really have so many and completely different conditions *or* is he suffering an allergic challenge to the various systems: eyes, nose, chest, etc.? You don't have to be Einstein to make the connection, yet it is often denied. It seems easier to ignore and keep referring than to look at the bigger picture and determine a structured management strategy.

Here's the unfortunate end result for many children.

- Many dermatologists refuse to accept a link between eczema and allergy even though it's screaming for attention.
- Many paediatricians refuse to do allergy tests, even where there is overwhelming evidence of a link between some sort of allergy and the presenting symptoms. ('Lift the carpets . . . get rid of the dog . . . try stopping milk' are some of the many speculative snippets of advice I've heard. Much money is spent on anti-allergy manoeuvres when the child doesn't have an allergy!)
- Expensive and inappropriate anti-asthma drugs are prescribed without any reference to the background cause triggering the response.

Perhaps the most baffling aspect of this is the indifference shown at all levels of the health system. With statistics suggesting that so many of the population have some type of allergy, there are more resources devoted to cardiovascular and osteoporosis screening programmes and suchlike than to providing even a minimal allergy service. It's disappointing to say the least.

This takes me back to the hay fever epidemic. Two hundred years ago the illness was unheard of and there is no one theory that explains the rise since. Conventional explanations simply do not fit the facts. Some scientists believe there may be a link between hay fever and other 'modern plagues' such as asthma and eczema.

For decades, those with hay fever have been led to believe that their condition is brought on by the amount of pollen in the air. When as few as 50 pollen grains per cubic yard of air are recorded it's classified as a 'high' pollen count, enough to trigger symptoms. Pollen is counted using a sampling device that is typically placed on a rooftop several storeys above the ground. The device has a sticky surface that collects grains of pollen from the air. Since pollen is so easily spread over a wide area, a sampling taken in one area is usually considered valid for a large area, even an entire city.

In the UK there is a National Pollen Research Unit and pollen levels have been studied here for many years. For example, levels in the mid 1970s were very high. They peaked in the summer of 1976 (and I remember it well, blissfully long hot and sunny summer days). In more recent decades pollen levels actually fell, reflecting the amount of grassland in Britain that was in decline, but since 2008 there's been a 'spectacular' increase. The Research Unit believes this could be related to climate change – particularly to milder temperatures in spring. In the last few years the UK and Ireland has had more than its usual share of rainfall in May. This has been followed by good weather in June – coinciding with the flowering season (Ireland had an especially wet June in 2012, bucking this trend).

However, allergists believe there are other factors than varying pollen counts to explain the surge in people with hay fever symptoms. They suggest the present epidemic may reflect a number of different interrelated issues.

Air pollution

This is one possible culprit. Hay fever was virtually unknown before the nineteenth century, despite far more of the countryside being under agricultural cultivation then, but there were no cars in those days. So, could exhaust fumes be contributing to the hay fever crisis? Well, pollution from cars has been linked to the parallel rise in asthma across Europe and North America. It is possible that particles in car exhaust fumes irritate the airways of certain susceptible people, leaving them more prone to both hay fever and asthma. Japan's experience helps us better understand this.

Known colloquially as 'kafunsho' (花粉症), nasal allergy is one of the most common diseases in Japan. Estimates suggest that anywhere from 15 to 30 per cent of Japan's population suffers from hay fever. The pollen from that country's *sugi* trees is high in the air between mid February and late April. Then the pollen from the *hinoki* trees lasts from early April to about mid May. That's a good three months of pollen-induced discomfort for those with tree-pollen allergy. However, Japanese citizens are mainly allergic to cedar tree pollen. Between the 1950s and the 1970s, around four and a half million hectares of cedar trees were planted in an attempt to meet the growing need for construction material in Japan. It eventually became more economical to import timber, which soon made the cedar plantations obsolete. As the cedar forests matured, the amount of cedar pollen in the air increased and the number of people with hay fever multiplied. A fascinating study also showed that both adults and children who lived close to motorways suffered more severe hay fever than their rural cousins. That's when the idea was formed of diesel fumes leaching particulate matter and linking with pollen grains to produce 'super-pollen', a more aggressive type of allergic troublemaker than ordinary pollen alone.

Here's another theory.

Better recognition of symptoms

Another plausible explanation is that we are more aware of what are and what are not allergic conditions (although that information hasn't filtered down to a number of doctors). A hundred years ago, serious diseases like measles, typhoid and tuberculosis were a fact of life for most families. With no National Health Service, people were reluctant to pay to see a doctor for anything other than the most serious conditions.

It seems likely an illness that – although unpleasant – was not life-threatening would have been dismissed by most people as not worth reporting. The modern tendency to over-diagnose every vague symptom as a named disease has almost certainly contributed to the rise in hay fever statistics, as it has done with other modern conditions such as autism and attention deficit disorder. But even when the over-reporting is taken into account, there is still a definite increase in the prevalence of hay fever worldwide or, more accurately, in 'Westernized' countries (there's more on this later in this chapter).

Over-exposure to antibiotics

Over the past 40 years, as widespread antibiotic use has climbed, so too have allergy rates. Have we unwittingly lulled our immune systems into 'off mode' by not allowing them to develop in response to bacteria and viruses? Then, as if annoyed by this inactivity, our immunity takes it out by overreacting to allergy challenge. It's an interesting concept and I feel it's a definite runner. Doctors did hand out antibiotics like jelly beans as each new product became available. The pharmaceutical industry encouraged this (putting profit before science). But this lazy medical approach has left us with a different health crisis – allergy. I recall that the most widely prescribed medicine in the late 1970s and early 1980s was a particular antibiotic called Amoxycillin. Ten years or so later the top prescribed drug was Salbutamol, used to treat asthma. Maybe that shift in the prescribing trend tells us something about doctors' attitudes to changing disease – and in what way these diseases were evolving. Was all that 'bronchitis' of the 1970s and 1980s really bronchitis (a chest infection) or was it really asthma (and allergy driven)? Did we miss the big picture completely? I *know* we did.

Finally, here's another concept to consider.

The hygiene hypothesis

This idea would appear to turn conventional wisdom on its head. But if it's correct it might explain all the increases in allergies seen in recent decades.

The theory is simple; allergies are on the rise because we are too clean. The idea that cleanliness is bad for you has crossed from folklore into mainstream immunology and is being taken increasingly seriously because scientists have been at such a loss to explain the increase in conditions like hay fever. In our sanitized, disinfected world, where every kitchen surface is sterile and our food is vacuum packed and cleansed of all germs, our immune systems are simply not getting the 'priming' they need to develop properly in infancy.

As a result, our bodies fail to distinguish between harmless dust or pollen and nasty bacteria that could kill and mount an unnecessary attack. By depriving our immune system of contact with key infections caused by viruses, bacteria and parasites, we fail to develop the necessary tolerance for ordinary, tame foreign particles. The immune system – underused and spoiling for a fight – goes overboard when finally given the opportunity, no matter how slight the opponent.

Poor people living in developing countries exhibit markedly

lower levels of allergy. This holds true even for impoverished communities within polluted urban centres. Dirt, in other words, may be good for you. But poor people living in developing countries can become allergic when they move to a more developed area. So parents who try to prevent their children coming into contact with any germs at all may be storing up problems for their offspring in later life.

Moreover, those living in Westernized countries tend to create more allergy-rich environments. Those of you who've read my previous book, *Sinusitis: Steps to healing* (Sheldon Press, 2009), may remember the case of 24-year-old Abasiofun Radigan, who lived in rural Nigeria where her lifestyle was simple. She shared a house made of concrete blocks and that had a thatched roof with her family. There were no carpets or curtains and minimal furniture. There were animals in the neighbourhood, cattle and dogs especially, but no domestic pets. Abasiofun was healthy, but, when she started working in Ireland in 2007, she developed severe head colds and sneezing attacks within a month. She had difficulty sleeping at night, was noticeably breathless with exertion and developed wheeziness and laboured breathing. Her skin, once smooth and unblemished, was now itchy and irritable.

By the time she had lived for 12 weeks in the country house where she worked, Abasiofun was so unwell she had to visit the local doctor. He recognized that the young woman had a severe nasal allergy that was triggering asthma. He also noticed she was developing eczema (itchy skin) in the areas usually seen in children, the creases of the knees and elbows. As part of her check-up, the doctor ordered allergy tests. The results showed that Abasiofun was severely allergic to horsehair, dust mites and cat hair – the owners of the house kept horses, dogs and cats. Minute particles, smaller than a speck of dust, of these allergy-provoking substances had swept inside the girl's nose and sinuses, triggering an aggressive nasal allergy. This in turn kick-started asthma and, slowly but gradually, eczema.

Abasiofun left the country house. In fact she left Ireland, too, and returned to her native Nigeria and better health.

Abasiofun must have been carrying the genetic code for allergy all her life. However, her basic living conditions and lifestyle in

Nigeria did not challenge her immune system and so she stayed well. The move to a damper and colder climate was a shock to her system. An even greater jolt was the amount of allergy-provoking material she suddenly became exposed to. Her immunity was challenged like never before and she started showing all the signs of a highly allergic individual. She first developed a nasal allergy (almost like hay fever), then asthma and finally eczema. (In babies such allergic events occur in the reverse order: i.e., eczema, followed by nasal allergy and eventually asthma.)

For most hay fever sufferers, moving to a low-allergy climate isn't an option. If Abasiofun's story highlights anything (and graphically, too), it's that some sufferers have both complicated and complex allergy problems.

10

Nasal lavage in hay fever

A better way to keep your nose and sinuses healthy

Blowing your nose to relieve the stuffiness caused by hay fever may be second nature, but some specialists in ear, nose and throat disorders argue it reverses the flow of mucus into the sinuses. It also slows the natural drainage of the sinuses.

To test the concept, infectious disease investigators at the University of Virginia in the USA conducted CT scans and other measurements as subjects coughed, sneezed and blew their noses. In some cases, the subjects had opaque dye dripped into their rear nasal cavities.

Coughing and sneezing generated little if any pressure in the nasal cavities. But nose blowing generated enormous pressure – 'equivalent to a person's blood pressure reading', one researcher said – and propelled mucus into the sinuses every time. The same doctor said it was unclear whether this was harmful, but added that during illness it could shoot viruses or bacteria into the sinuses and possibly cause further infection.

Conclusion: blowing your nose can create a build-up of excess pressure in the sinus cavities.

According to experts in the Ear, Nose and Throat Department at the New York University Langone Medical Centre, the correct method is to blow one nostril at a time and to take decongestants. This prevents a build-up of excess pressure. So what do you do if you're troubled with nose problems and experts warn against that most traditional of remedies for relief, blowing the nose? You should consider nasal lavage (also known as nasal irrigation, nasal douching or sinus rinsing).

The principle of sinus irrigation

While some level of mucus production from the nasal and sinus lining is normal, allergies (such as hay fever) and sinus infections can cause excessive mucus production. This excess mucus causes nasal and sinus symptoms such as a runny and stuffy nose or post-nasal drip. The key to symptom relief is to physically wash away from the nasal passages this excess mucus and the associated allergens, such as grass and tree pollens, dust particles, pollutants and bacteria. Rinsing in this way will reduce inflammation of the nasal membrane, allowing you to breathe more normally. In summary, nasal lavage:

- gets rid of any allergy-provoking material in your nose, including pollens;
- gets rid of any pockets of infection that might be forming;
- clears your nose and makes it easier to breathe;
- moisturizes your nasal lining;
- feels refreshing.

All that's involved is squirting a solution of slightly salty water up your nose, letting it drip out, blowing your nose gently, then repeating. The mechanical action of flushing out thickened mucus cleanses the nasal passages, making it easier for the cilia, the tiny hair-like structures that line the nose, to push the remaining mucus out.

There is strong support for nasal lavage among allergists and ENT specialists. 'Many patients who have sinus disease, allergies, or chronic infections are improved tremendously by lavaging their nose out once or twice a day,' says a top USA-based ENT specialist. 'And for those who have had surgery to open up narrowed sinuses, regular cleansing is a must. The main improvement they experience is the ability to wash out the cavity.'

'Even if antibacterial medications are added to the lavage solution, most of the benefit is from the mechanical rinsing of the nasal cavity,' says yet another ENT specialist at the Massachusetts Eye and Ear Infirmary. 'Among other things, the gunk you rinse out in mucus includes natural chemicals called cytokines, which promote inflammation. If you remove the mucus, you can actually reduce the inflammation.' He emphasizes that the way to do this is with salty water.

While large, controlled studies of nasal lavage for treating and preventing colds and sinus infections are hard to come by, the little data that does exist seems to support the practice. One study of more than 200 patients published in 2000 in the journal *Laryngoscope* found that after three to six weeks of nasal irrigation, patients reported statistically fewer nasal symptoms. A 1997 study of 21 volunteers in the same journal found that lavage improved the speed with which nasal cilia were able to move mucus along. A 1998 study in children published in the *Journal of Allergy and Clinical Immunology* showed that lavage is 'tolerable, inexpensive, and effective'.

Effective nasal irrigation devices must have the following:

- the capacity to hold a large volume of saline solution (200 to 240 ml);
- the ability to deliver the solution with low but adequate pressure into the nasal passages (the pressure must be sufficient that the saline can not only flow through the nasal passages, but also displace the mucus, pollen and other allergens);
- finally, the saline solution must travel up the nasal passage and

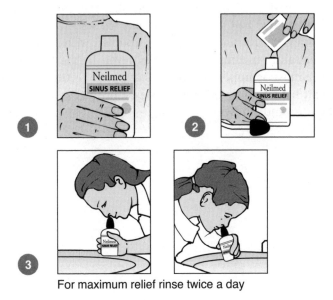

For maximum relief rinse twice a day

Figure 10.1 Sinus irrigation

out through the other nostril – unless this entire flow cycle occurs, you may not achieve a thorough cleansing job.

Neilmed Sinus Rinse ticks all the boxes for success. It's essentially a plastic squeeze bottle that holds 240 ml of liquid. With it come small sachets that contain salt and baking soda granules in an isotonic combination ideal for nasal irrigation. To use, you boil a kettle of water and let the water cool until it is just warm. Empty one sachet into the squeeze bottle and top up with the warm water to the level on the side. Make sure the granules are dissolved. At the top of the black cap on the bottle is an opening. This is held against one nostril opening (see Figure 10.1), with your head slightly tilted forward over a wash basin. Squeeze the bottle firmly: one half of the contents should go up one nostril and come down the other side. Pause, blow the nose gently and repeat the procedure on the opposite nostril. This washes the nose and sinuses clean, and clears snotty debris as well as allergens such as tree and grass pollens, bacteria, viruses, etc. that may be lurking on the nasal lining. The salt and baking soda combination is remarkably refreshing for those with sinusitis and they are delighted with the non-medical components of the product.

Nasal irrigation is more or less the mainstay of treatment for people who have had sinus surgery, but it's something to recommend as a daily routine for anyone troubled with nasal issues of whatever cause, including pollen hay fever. In the USA, it's considered almost as important as brushing your teeth and combing your hair before going out for the day. Consider it as dental floss for the nose and sinuses.

11

Non-medical hay fever remedies

I'm pretty much an orthodox doctor who uses standard medicines to help my patients. I'm also long enough in the tooth to know that many of them don't like taking medicines (and in truth I'm not a big fan of prescribing them), but there is a life choice trade-off with medical ailments. Do you want to suffer or would you rather take something to make you feel better? Do you want to fight that chest infection with honey and lemon or take an antibiotic to clear it up? At what point do you decide to drop the honey and lemon plan, bite the bullet and ask your doctor for help? In my experience that's often when the bacteria have moved to the lungs. It's no longer a simple chest infection; rather it's become life-threatening pneumonia. If so, that is *not* the time to be looking for alternative remedies to pull you back to good health.

In 2003, when it looked as if the leukaemia I'd been battling for four years was going to win, I had no option but to take chemotherapy and immunotherapy. I didn't particularly want to take these drugs, but I had a simple, stark choice: take the treatment or die within six months. Since I was in my early fifties, I decided I was too young to die – especially as I had a wife and two young children to support. I signed up for the programme like a drowning man reaching for a life belt. As I told the oncology nurse, 'If I have to perform handstands naked in Dublin's O'Connell Street to stay alive I'll do it.'

Fortunately for the good citizens of Dublin, that wasn't necessary. Instead I was hooked up to green bags containing drugs that dripped into a vein in my arm. Written in large letters on each bag was: DANGEROUS. IF THIS SPILLS CLEAR THE AREA AND NOTIFY STAFF. CONTENTS MUST BE CLEANED BY TRAINED PERSONNEL. And all the time it was dripping into my bloodstream. Bundle of fun, eh? Medicine so dangerous it could clear a whole ward if spilled, and here I was, lapping it up so to speak. But it worked, and I'm still walking, talking and chewing gum. And writing books.

As well as anti-cancer drugs, many in the ward also took herbal, homeopathic and alternative medicine remedies. They believed in helping the body fight cancer naturally by boosting the immune system. I don't know whether those who used alternative remedies fared any better than me, but I understood their desire to do everything and anything to help them recover.

Hay fever will not kill you but it does make life miserable. So, for those who do prefer to use alternative medicines, either exclusively or to supplement their other treatments, then the following strategies and compounds are the best I'm aware of. All the following information comes from reputable and experienced alternative medical practitioners. Most of the words are theirs, so you may notice significant variations in explanations from what you've read so far. I hope you find something here to help you with your hay fever.

Honey

Taking the honey bees make from pollen doesn't add to the woes of people with hay fever. Some herbalists believe honey's stickiness helps to coat the lining of the throat and soothe the soreness that hay fever brings about. Others say that small amounts of reactive pollen help to desensitize the user and build up some immunity by the time the summer months come around (which is very much like the immunotherapy treatment I described in Chapter 5).

The person with hay fever takes two tablespoons of honey every day three months before the hay fever season kicks in. While honey contains traces of pollen, it doesn't give you hay fever or worsen hay fever symptoms. This is because honey is made from heavy-grained pollens that don't trigger allergies. Honey is also cited as having more effective antibacterial and healing properties than many of the usual over-the-counter solutions, and it certainly tastes a lot better. Thousands of people swear by their spoonfuls of honey a day, be it Manuka, heather honey, floral honey or simple filtered and pasteurized honey. So maybe there is something in that sticky syrup that helps soothe the itchiness of a hay fever attack.

What type of honey?
Most people recommend honey made by bees close to the area where you live. This is based on the principle that you're more likely to be allergic to local pollen than distant pollen. So find a source from a local farmer or beekeeper.

A spokesperson from the Honey Association says any neighbourhood product could work. 'Honey isn't a processed product. All we do is strain it to take out the impurities and heat it gently to 40–50° C to get it into jars. Straining shouldn't matter as the strainer holes are much bigger than the pollen. Heating wouldn't kill off the pollen, which is very robust – you can still find honey in ancient Egyptian tombs. And it makes no difference whether the honey is clear or set, that's just how it crystallizes.'

Will honey definitely help my hay fever?
This depends on which pollens you're allergic to and whether or not these have been used by the bees making your local honey. For example, you might suffer from allergies to tree and grass pollens, while the honey you buy has only tree pollens in it. This might help reduce your reactivity to tree pollens at the beginning of the summer but leave you vulnerable to the bigger grass pollen challenge a month or so later. If the honey contains traces of tree *and* grass pollens, you might be spared both. It all depends on which mixture of pollen grains your local bees buzz around when drawing their nectar.

Honey is not a cure for hay fever. It has worked for thousands of people and disappointed as many others. I suggest you ignore the snide comments from ultra-conservative medics who delight in saying, 'There is no proven study to show honey has any effect in curing hay fever symptoms.' It's definitely worth a try. No matter how it might work it'll certainly do no harm.

Somebody said I have to swallow it raw. Is that true?
Honey is honey, whether you swallow two tablespoons outright or mix it into an exotic concoction. So how you swallow it doesn't matter. Some herbalists suggest putting three tablespoons of honey into a cup of nettle tea. They say nettle tea is a natural antihistamine and clears excess mucus in the respiratory system. Alternatively, you might want to mix it with lemon juice or even bake it into a scrumptious cake! If the honey has solidified in places, simply heat it in some warm water to liquefy it.

Possible side effects

Honey contains salicylates (see 'Diet', opposite), which some people are sensitive to. Since honey is clammy, it may attract small quantities of lighter wind-blown pollens from outside. This could trigger inflammation of the nasal lining and eyes. However, such plants only bloom around late April, so it's safe to use honey before that. But don't overdo it. I don't want you hay fever free but as fat as a fool by September.

Garlic

Another, less sweet hay fever alternative is the vampire's nemesis: garlic. This antioxidant has a wealth of positive health effects including antibacterial, antiviral and antifungal properties. It even helps cholesterol levels. Regular consumption of garlic is thought to boost your immune system while also providing a natural anti-inflammatory and antihistamine effect, as it contains quercetin (a plant-derived flavonoid found in fruit, vegetables, leaves and grains). Garlic's healing properties are best absorbed when ingested crushed or raw, which might not ingratiate you with your social circle. To prevent the dreaded bad breath associated with garlic, opt for garlic capsules which you can buy at any pharmacy.

Acupuncture

If you have an interest in Chinese medicine or you have previously benefited from acupuncture, then this may be the treatment for you. While many of us don't relish having needles inserted into our faces, there are many others who get great relief from this technique. Acupuncture can be used in particular to relieve the runny nose and itchy eyes that plague those with hay fever. It is recommended to have between four and six sessions before the hay fever season begins in order to get the best results, but this is not guaranteed. Some people will find that acupuncture can all but rid them of the symptoms that have ruined their summers for years; for others there will be no noticeable benefit.

Vaseline

This is one of the less attractive options for those with hay fever but it undoubtedly helps to produce a barrier method against those pesky allergens. Smearing a thin layer of Vaseline on the insides of the lower nostrils can help to trap pollen particles that are attempting to make their way into your airways and prevent inflammation symptoms from worsening. However, it is a fair trade-off; a glistening nose without an itch or a run surely trumps the allergic alternative. Try the aloe vera version to soothe your over-wiped nostrils.

Diet

If you are prone to food sensitivities or food-related allergies, then these could be interlinked with your hay fever symptoms. For some people the identification of problematic foods and ingredients can help to relieve or reduce hay fever symptoms. Food groups such as dairy can cause extra congestion in some people. Remember that if you're allergic to birch pollen you may also react to celery, curry spices, raw tomato, raw carrot, apples, pears and kiwi fruit. If you're allergic to grass pollen you may also react to oats, rye, wheat, kiwi fruit and raw tomato. If your allergy is to weed pollen you may also react to raw carrots and curry spices.

If you have hay fever with diminished senses of smell and taste and you erupt in hives occasionally, then avoid the following *salicylate*-containing foods and the specific food additives mentioned earlier (this is explained in greater detail in Chapter 8). Salicylates (a set of chemicals that occur naturally but are also manufactured for their health properties; unfortunately some people are exquisitely allergic to them) are found in certain foods and, depending on how troublesome your sinusitis is, you may be told to avoid these foods totally or, more likely, advised to consume them in small quantities only. Do not mix and match throughout this group such that you might unwittingly consume large quantities. The foods are:

dried fruits	pineapples
berry fruits	cucumbers
oranges	gherkins
apricots	tomato sauce

tea	liquorice
endives	peppermints
olives	honey (as mentioned above)
grapes	Worcestershire sauce
almonds	

Many spices also contain high salicylate levels.

When taste becomes impaired in hay fever the sensation of spice is the first to go. Adults and children who find their sense of taste impaired tend to look for tangier, spicier foods and flavourings. Unfortunately almost all tang and spice is artificially created using chemicals. Those with hay fever can unwittingly make their condition worse (and add in an extra problem) by using artificially flavoured foods, especially in Indian and Chinese dishes.

There are many chemical additives used by the food and drink industry and by law the manufacturer must inform the consumer what compounds are in the can or tin or packet. The additives are used to colour, flavour or preserve food and drinks. For example, if you buy a packet of cheese and onion crisps, there's neither cheese nor onion in the product: the taste is created by using artificial flavourings. When you reach for a brightly coloured fizzy drink on the supermarket shelf, more often than not the colour is also artificially created. Some foods and drinks have all three types of chemicals in them: colourings, flavourings and preservatives. Because the chemicals have long and strange-sounding names the industry works to a code. Nowadays each additive is labelled by number and with the letter E attached (known as 'E numbers').

So, as part of your overall management, you should avoid the food additives listed in Chapter 8, especially E621, monosodium glutamate. Where there is poor labelling or the phrase 'contains permitted additives' or 'contains permitted colourings and flavourings' or just says 'colourings and flavourings', it's best to avoid the product. Indeed, it's best to avoid any product coloured red, orange, yellow, blue, lemon or green, as there is a strong chance it will contain one of the listed agents. Check tablets, capsules, lozenges, vitamin preparations and even the stripes in toothpaste. If you are unsure about the safety of a product, avoid it.

A low histamine diet

The following foods and drinks contain high levels of histamine. Active hay fever releases histamine into the bloodstream and that triggers a lot of hay fever symptoms. So don't add to your histamine load by consuming foods or drinks rich in the compound. The following products should be avoided as part of your overall management:

- *fish*: tuna, sardine, anchovy, mackerel
- *cheese*: Emmenthal, Harzer, Gouda, Roquefort, Tilsiter, Camembert, Cheddar
- *hard, cured sausages*, including salami and dried ham
- *vegetables*: pickled cabbage, spinach, tomatoes and tomato ketchup
- *alcohol*: red wine (especially deep and heavy reds), white wine, sparkling wine, beer.

Omega-3 fatty acids

These may act to lower the amounts of inflammatory chemicals produced by the body after exposure to an allergen. Although additional research is needed, it appears that a diet high in omega-3 fatty acids may help decrease the incidence of hay fever.

Changing your off-licence choices

Alcohol can worsen hay fever symptoms due to the yeast and bacteria that are part of the fermentation process. Sulphites in wines also intensify hay fever (and many other allergy problems). For most of us, though, staying away from alcohol all summer just isn't an option, so the next best thing is to stick to the beverages that have less chance of making your nose run. In this case it's spirits such as vodka, which contain less histamine and contribute less to your allergies than beer and wine, but don't become a drunken sot trying to cope with hay fever!

'Word of mouth' remedies

Chicken soup and lemon

Some researchers believe there are anti-inflammatory properties in chicken soup. So a 'soup and lemon juice' combination may help by reducing dehydration, mucus production and nasal congestion.

Vodka steam

Boil ½ pint of water and add a shot of vodka. Put the combination in a large bowl, cover your head with a towel and inhale the vapours. Maybe it's the soporific effect of the alcohol vapour that helps, but patients, especially those from eastern Europe, swear by this remedy.

Vitamin C tablets in a cup of tea

Vitamin C is everyone's go-to vitamin when it comes to colds and flu, but it shouldn't be overlooked as a source of antihistamine during the hay fever season. High doses of vitamin C (250–500 mg, taken three times a day) may ease inflammation in the mucous membranes and can be taken in capsules. If you want to source your vitamin C naturally, then stock up on fruit like strawberries, blueberries and raspberries, which contain bioflavonoids that help the body to retain and absorb the vitamin C. Vegetables such as broccoli, cabbage, brussels sprouts, kale, turnips, spinach and peppers also contain high levels of vitamin C. The antioxidants in vitamin C help modulate your immune reaction to viral head colds. And a cup of tea perks you up.

Milk and garlic

Garlic is an antioxidant and anti-inflammatory agent, so it might help for those reasons alone.

Camomile steam baths

These are worth trying; inhale the camomile from a bowl with a cloth over the head. Other ethereal oils, for instance eucalyptus, pine tree, fir and peppermint, also reduce swelling of the mucous membranes and dissolve secretion congestions. These oils should not be used when you are being treated with homeopathic remedies.

Homeopathy

Homeopathy is a form of complementary healthcare that works with our natural healing process and has been successfully used for over 200 years. The word comes from the Greek and means 'similar suffering'. This refers to its central philosophy that a substance which produces symptoms in a healthy person can cure those symptoms in a sick person. For example, someone with hay fever might be given the remedy *Allium cepa* (prepared from an onion), because a healthy person chopping an onion usually experiences watering eyes and irritation. However, the substances are given in minute doses prepared in a specific way to prevent unwanted side effects, making them safe to use where conventional drugs would be dangerous or inadvisable (e.g. during pregnancy or when treating infants).

Homeopathy practitioners say their phones never stop ringing during the pollen season. So here are their top hay fever tips. These recommendations are based on what symptoms the patient is suffering. For a more comprehensive assessment, consult a qualified and experienced practitioner.

Homeopathic tree and grass pollen mix

This is a bit like immunotherapy, as described in Chapter 5. Here a combination of pollens from plants, trees and various grasses are swallowed in daily capsules prior to and throughout the pollen season.

Allium cepa, sabadilla and euphrasia

These are first-line hay fever remedies and improve irritated eyes and nose.

Allium cepa is used when the symptoms are mainly strong burning sensations from the nose and eyes, accompanied by a watery discharge. The eyes are sensitive to light, often red and irritated, while the nose can become red and sore from the burning, corrosive mucus. There can be violent sneezing, the voice can be hoarse and there can be a hacking cough. The kind of hay fever that is best tackled with *Allium cepa* often comes in spring or August and is made worse by being in a warm room, improving in cool air. One peculiarity of this remedy is that it particularly affects the left eye or nostril, or may start off on the left side and spread to the right.

Sabadilla is most often indicated during early spring or at harvest time. Then there can be persistent sneezing, transparent mucus and an itchy, stuffed-up nose. The eyes may water in the open air from sunlight or while sneezing. Symptoms are also worse in cold air, and there is usually improvement from eating warm food and warm drinks or by keeping warm.

Euphrasia has a long history of use in herbalism for eye conditions, so it is no surprise that its main homeopathic use is for conditions that seem to centre on the eyes. It is useful for very watery eyes, when the person may feel the need to wipe or rub them constantly. The eyelids (particularly the lower eyelids) can swell up and there can be a thick, infected discharge from the eye itself. There can be the sensation of a foreign body (such as a grain of sand) in the eyes and they can become very gummed up and sore. The nasal and throat symptoms are less marked but include watery mucus that is easily discharged. Euphrasia cures symptoms that occur in sunlight or windy weather, and indoors.

Euphrasia tincture can also be used as a local eyewash by diluting one drop in an eyebath of cooled sterile water. It is very soothing for sore eyes at any time.

Arsenicum

This is indicated in people who have frequent sneezing and a blocked nose accompanied by a watery discharge. Unlike *Allium cepa* it treats symptoms that are worse outside and improve if the person can stay in the house and keep warm. The eyes may be inflamed, with burning and swelling that is somewhat relieved by warm bathing. The right side is generally more affected than the left and there can be a marked worsening of symptoms during the night, particularly when lying down. Generally the person requiring Arsenicum may feel unduly restless or anxious during the attack and find it difficult to get warm – even in hot weather.

Arundo

This is useful when the hay fever begins with burning and itching of the palate and eyes or if there's an annoying itch in the nostrils.

Ferrum phos

Very useful in the early stages of any inflammation. Taken when allergy symptoms start, it often slows or stops an episode. Use when symptoms include runny eyes with a burning or gritty feeling, facial flushing, watery nose and short, hard, tickling cough.

Natrum muriaticum

Take when the nasal discharge has the consistency of raw egg white. The catarrh is usually white or clear and watery and can be extremely profuse. There is often repeated violent sneezing – especially in the mornings – a loss of smell or taste and itching in the nose. The eyes can be watery and the throat can be dry and sore. Any nasal allergy responding to this remedy can often be accompanied by violent, pulsating headaches made much worse by the heat of the sun or by increased physical or emotional activity. The patient may prefer to be alone and feel quite touchy or tearful. In some cases cold sores can develop around the nose or lips. Symptoms are worse with heat or when lying down. They improve with cold showers, at the seashore or in the open air.

Nux vomica

One of the main themes indicating use of this remedy is 'irritability', which can be apparent on the physical or emotional level. People who need this may be cross or oversensitive and have acute sensitivity to the slightest odour or particle of pollen. There can be a very stuffed-up nose in alternating nostrils, intense itching of the ears, nose and eyes, and the unsatisfied urge to sneeze. The face can be very hot but the body often feels cold. The throat can feel rough and dry and, if the hay fever continues, the person may experience queasiness. This is one remedy to think of particularly if there has been a bad reaction to antihistamine drugs that caused a disordered liver or digestion. Symptoms are worse in the morning, when stimulants such as coffee or alcohol have been consumed, when there are strong smells in the vicinity or if the person is angry. A short sleep, eating or a warm drink may bring about improvement.

Pulsatilla

Try this when thick green catarrh is produced from the eyes and nose. The catarrh can become obstructed and lead to sinusitis, nosebleeds or a loss of smell, although it is often more fluid in the open air. There is a sensation of burning and dryness in the eyes and the lids can become gummed up, with styes forming. Generally those who respond to Pulsatilla are emotionally more sensitive, irritable or tearful, with changing moods. Their physical and emotional states can also be very changeable from day to day. Symptoms are normally worse in the evenings, in the sun, and better with cold applications and in cool, fresh air.

Sulphur

Used when there's a lot of thick, offensive catarrh. The person may generally feel hot and symptoms may be aggravated if he or she becomes too hot. The nose and eyes can become inflamed, with heat and burning sensations. There can be oversensitivity to odours or changes in temperature. Classically this type of hay fever may be accompanied by a skin rash or by itching anywhere on the body. The throat may become swollen and the person may be far hungrier than usual. Symptoms are worse with bathing or in the late morning and improve with exercise and fresh air.

Sanguinaria

This is prepared from a herb that occurs naturally in the United States, Canada and India. It goes by the common name of *Bloodroot*. Medical complaints that can be treated by Sanguinaria include hay fever and asthma.

Wyethia

Often prescribed when there's an intolerable itching on the roof of the mouth and behind the nose, sometimes extending into the throat and ears. Everything in the head of the person with hay fever feels dry and irritated, but the nose may still be runny.

Royal jelly, ginseng and echinacea

Much success has been reported by those with hay fever (especially women in the menopause) on a daily regime of a formulation called *Irene*, which acts on the immune system. A natural substance without side effects, Irene is a blend of royal jelly, ginseng and echinacea. It was developed by Irene Stein, the woman who introduced royal jelly to the Western world in the 1970s.

Royal jelly has been used successfully in China for thousands of years to treat a wide range of ailments. Its success in a variety of conditions is attributed to its balancing effect on the immune system. Royal jelly is the food fed exclusively to the queen bee in the beehive and as a result she lives up to six times longer than the other bees and produces an astonishing 2,000 eggs a day. Almost like breast milk, royal jelly plays a key part in the nutrition of the queen bee. Possibly by providing enormous energy it may enhance her immunity.

Ginseng has also been in use in Chinese herbal medicines for centuries, as has echinacea. Put together in a single and accessible product, the benefits of Irene are 'slow but steady'.

Herbal remedies

Chinese herbs

Yin Chiao herbs may have antioxidant properties that help with immune stimulation and speed up recovery from hay fever. (Antioxidants are widely used as ingredients in dietary supplements in the hope of maintaining health and preventing diseases such as cancer and coronary heart disease. Although some studies have suggested antioxidant supplements have health benefits, other large clinical trials have not detected any benefit.)

Camomile

Camomile tea is reputed to relieve hay fever symptoms. Some herbalists suggest smearing camomile and lemon oil on a tissue and inhaling to relieve hay fever symptoms.

Ginger

Ginger tea and raw honey work to break up chest congestion and loosen phlegm. Ginger strengthens the immune system and acts as a natural antihistamine.

Green tea

This blocks the production of histamine and is one of the best homemade remedies for building the immune system.

Peppermint

Peppermint tea relieves nasal and sinus congestion. Drink it cold to soothe the coughing associated with hay fever and allergies.

Butterbur

Effective in reducing inflammation, blocking histamines and leukotrienes. Studies suggest the herb is effective for relieving sneezing, itchy eyes, sinus congestion and headaches. People allergic to ragweed or chrysanthemum should avoid butterbur.

Steaming

This produces excellent results to break up congestion. Add a few drops of eucalyptus oil to a bowl of hot water and carefully inhale the steam. Avoid eucalyptus if you are taking other homeopathic remedies as it may block their benefits.

Grapefruit and lemon

Boiled in one cup of water for 15 minutes, this makes an excellent home remedy for hay fever. Use only the flesh, not the rind. Cool and mix with raw honey to relieve symptoms.

Calendula

Liquid calendula diluted in water makes an excellent eye wash to soothe itchy eyes. Use non-alcoholic calendula. Add a dropper full of colloidal silver to enhance the antimicrobial action and reduce inflammation.

12

Cigarette smoking and hay fever

In Chapter 6 I advised readers not to bother with anti-allergy programmes if there is a smoker in the family. This is because *passive smoking aggravates all allergies*.

Here are a few facts about smoking and passive smoking. If you're reading this book it suggests that you hope to find an answer to your hay fever or that of your child. But if you or your child are around a smoker, then you might as well throw the book away, as the destructive effects of tobacco will more than outweigh any health measures you adopt.

About passive smoking

There is ample evidence to show that respiratory health in both children and adults suffers badly when they are exposed to cigarette smoke. Unless otherwise stated, statistics are from Action on Smoking and Health (ASH).

- The immediate effects of exposure to secondhand smoke include eye irritation, headache, cough, sore throat, dizziness and nausea. Adults with asthma may experience a significant decline in lung function when exposed, while new cases of asthma may be brought on in children whose parents smoke.
- As little as an hour of exposure to secondhand smoke can cause a dramatic decline in lung function. Longer exposure can induce asthma and progressive decline in lung function, and has a major role in causing chronic respiratory disease.
- Passive smoking is a cause of lung cancer and heart disease in adult non-smokers, and of respiratory disease, cot death, middle ear infections and asthma in children.
- In households where both parents smoke, young children have a 72 per cent increased risk of respiratory illnesses.

- Children who suffer from asthma, and whose parents smoke, are twice as likely to suffer asthma symptoms all year round compared to the children of non-smokers.
- Children who are regularly exposed to secondhand tobacco smoke when travelling by car have significantly higher rates of hay fever and wheezing than those without such exposure (according to a study from the Tobacco Free Research Institute, Dublin).
- In Victoria, Australia, it is illegal to smoke in cars carrying children under 18.

It is estimated that, globally, 600,000 deaths a year are caused by secondhand smoke. The British Medical Association says there is no safe level of exposure to secondhand smoke.

About smoking

If you're unlucky enough to smoke yourself, the facts are even starker.

- In Britain, 40 per cent of all cancer deaths are from lung cancer, which is very rare in non-smokers.
- Smoking causes more deaths from heart attacks than from lung cancer and bronchitis. Smokers have two or three times the risk of a fatal heart attack as non-smokers.
- About 40 per cent of all heavy smokers die before 65. Only 10 per cent of smokers reach 75 in reasonable health.
- Other cancers more common in smokers than in non-smokers include tongue, throat, larynx, pancreatic, kidney, bladder and cervical cancers.
- Smoking is even worse for people with diabetes, as it exacerbates the extra risks they face of heart disease, stroke and kidney disease.

How smoking affects the respiratory system

Tobacco smoke contains over 4,000 chemicals including carbon monoxide, arsenic, formaldehyde, cyanide and benzene.

Carbon monoxide

This gas takes the place of oxygen in the blood, so that less oxygen reaches the brain, heart, muscles and other organs. Carbon monoxide affects the ability of the red blood cells to carry oxygen round the body and leaves muscles slightly stiffer than normal. This includes the heart muscle – as well as having less oxygen, a heart affected by carbon monoxide will be less able to contract properly, thus pumping blood less efficiently.

Nicotine

This also affects blood flow by narrowing small arteries, leaving less room for the blood to move through them. Nicotine also raises levels of blood glucose and blood cholesterol, causing arteries to degenerate and raising the risk of stroke.

Tar

Tar, a carcinogen, is sticky and brown; it stains teeth, fingernails and lung tissue. Tar further reduces the ability of red cells to pick up oxygen and causes damage and scarring to the lungs.

Hydrogen cyanide

This prevents the natural lung clearance carried out by cilia that move foreign substances out. This means that the chemicals in tobacco smoke can build up inside the lungs.

Other chemicals that damage the lungs include hydrocarbons, nitrous oxides, organic acids, phenols and oxidizing agents. As a result, cigarette smoke:

- causes swelling and narrowing of the lung airways;
- results in excess mucus in the lung passages;
- reduces lung function and causes breathlessness;
- causes coughing and wheezing;
- irritates the windpipe (trachea) and voice box (larynx);
- increases the risk of lung infection;
- can cause permanent damage to the lungs' air sacs.

How to stop smoking

More than a million Britons have stopped smoking each year for the last 15 years, and only one in three adults now smokes. On average, people who eventually stop smoking have made three or four previous attempts. Don't give up. Get help if necessary.

Reasons to stop abound, but the motivation has to come from you. Once you've made the decision, there is plenty of help and advice around. A good place to start is ASH (Action on Smoking and Health) – its 15 top tips on stopping can be found at <http://www.ash.org.uk/files/documents/ASH_129.pdf>

ASH also recommends helplines and suggests ways to get professional help if you need it. Your doctor may also be able to help if you are having difficulty stopping. Stop Smoking clinics are available on the NHS or you may be given a prescription of Zyban if you are having trouble (which helps, like all aids to smoking cessation, but won't do all the work for you).

Tips for stopping smoking

Stop completely

Stop as if you had never smoked at all. Throw away all cigarettes and get rid of any smoking props, such as lighters or ashtrays. It's sometimes recommended that you set a date to stop, but whenever you do it, it's best to go cold turkey rather than cutting down gradually. Research shows that even if you smoke fewer cigarettes than usual, your nicotine levels remain nearly the same because you inhale more of each cigarette. Adherence to just one rule is an almost guarantee of success . . . *never take another puff.*

Nicotine rewired your brain, growing millions of nicotinic receptors in 11 different regions. Your mind's nicotine-induced dopamine/adrenalin intoxication is a chemical dependency and every bit as real and permanent as alcoholism. Treating a true addiction as though it were some nasty little habit is a recipe for relapse. There is no such thing as just one puff. Recovery from nicotine dependency truly is all or nothing.

Get support

Tell family and friends you're giving up – and if any other smokers will join you, it may make your effort easier.

Don't be frightened of withdrawal symptoms

People who have to stop smoking for medical reasons, because they have been admitted to hospital with heart problems, for example, tend not to have withdrawal symptoms, which suggests that these are psychological rather than physical. The desire to smoke is usually at its strongest for the first 12 to 24 hours after stopping, but subsides as levels of tobacco-related chemicals drop in your body and generally eases over two to four weeks. Some people have symptoms such as restlessness and irritability, headaches, anxiety and nausea. Some people find, to their surprise, that any cough gets worse – this is just the airways clearing, so don't be discouraged. One technique for coping with cravings is to practise slow, deep breathing while clearing your mind of all needless chatter by focusing on your favourite person, place or thing. Another is to say your ABC, associating each letter with your favourite food, person or place. For example, 'A' is for apple pie, 'B' for your favourite beach, etc. It's doubtful you'll reach the end of the alphabet.

Be aware of smoking situations

Be prepared for psychological cravings in smoking-related situations, such as at social events, especially those involving alcohol.

Give yourself time to get used to your new habits

Allow a day, a week and then a month.

Prepare for emotional crises

Chemical dependency on nicotine is one of the most intense, repetitive and dependable relationships you're ever likely to know. Prepare to experience a normal sense of emotional loss when quitting.

Weight gain

Everyone worries about this. Narrow your focus on to giving up tobacco first. Try to avoid foods that contain sugar and fat. It may help to nibble on apples and carrots to give your hands and mouth something to do while breaking the smoking habit.

Don't skip meals

Each cigarette allowed you to skip meals without experiencing hunger pangs. Don't add needless symptoms to withdrawal, but instead learn to spread your normal daily calorie intake out more evenly over the entire day. Don't eat more food, but eat less food more often. Drink plenty of acidic fruit juice during the first three days. Cranberry juice is excellent and a bottle will cost you about the same as a pack of cigarettes. It will help both to accelerate the 72 hours or so needed to remove the alkaloid nicotine from your body and stabilize blood sugars. Take care beyond three days, as juices can be fattening.

Prepare for smoking dreams

Many successful cigarette quitters recall extremely vivid smoking dreams. It's actually a good sign, suggesting you're beginning to ease the need for cigarettes into your subconscious and then beyond, hopefully for good.

Smoking aids

They are just that – aids, not infallible remedies. They work to support your determined decision to give up – but they can't make that decision for you.

Aids include nicotine replacement therapy, which comes as gums, sprays, patches, tablets, lozenges and inhalers, which can be bought over the counter. Other methods include acupuncture, hypnosis, self-help groups and books, counselling and audio CDs.

Finally, don't give up. The payback both in health and in money in your pocket is worth any personal hell you may go through. No pain, no gain.

13

Hay fever and the menopause

Hormones and the body's immune system are close friends. Like a delicate lace web, their relationship can easily be disturbed or damaged. Keeping that in mind, it's not surprising when the female body goes through hormonal transitions such as puberty, menstruation, pregnancy or, in this case, menopause, allergies and other immune problems kick in.

As the menopause approaches, a woman's body prepares for life without menstruation. The main female hormones (oestrogen and progesterone) start to drop, slowly at first but then dramatically as the ovaries close down and cease production of these natural chemicals. Hormone fluctuations have a major impact on the start of allergy symptoms and the severity of the symptoms. Although why and how this happens is not fully understood, changes in hormone levels are frequently associated with the development of such allergic conditions as asthma, hay fever and eczema. Along with hormonal causes of allergies, other factors can trigger increased susceptibility to allergies or intensified symptoms. Some of those factors include diet, some types of medications and stress. Perimenopausal women who haven't had a period for six months experience as much as an 80 per cent increase in respiratory symptoms for conditions such as hay fever and asthma compared to non-menopausal women.

The best way to assure relief is to understand this link between allergy and waning hormones. And what treatment strategies are available.

About allergies

Allergies surface when your immune system reacts abnormally to foreign substances that are typically harmless to most people. Perhaps the most common example (especially since this is a book on hay fever) is an allergy to grass pollen.

When a woman is allergic, her immune system mistakenly identifies the substance as harmful. In an overreaction, so as to 'self-protect', it produces an allergic reaction, releasing IgE antibodies. These spark reactions that discharge histamine into the bloodstream. Histamine causes swelling and irritability of the tissue involved. The end results (in hay fever) are those familiar symptoms of sneezing, runny nose, blocked nose, watery, red and itchy eyes.

Types of allergy

Just to recap, many people have allergies to animal fur and dander, pollen and certain types of food, but, really, almost anything can be a cause of allergy.

- *Hay fever* is the most common of the allergic diseases and refers to seasonal nasal symptoms due to pollen.
- *Asthma* is a breathing problem that results from the inflammation and spasm of the lung's air passages.
- *Allergic eyes* is inflammation of the tissue layers that cover the surface of the eyeball and the under surface of the eyelid.
- *Allergic eczema* is an allergic rash of the skin. It's often associated with hay fever and asthma.
- *Hives* are skin reactions that appear as itchy swellings and can occur on any part of the body.
- *Allergic shock* is a life-threatening allergic reaction that can affect a number of organs at the same time. This response typically occurs when the allergen is eaten (for example foods) or injected (for example a bee sting).

The body's hormones and immune system use many of the same chemical messengers that trigger allergy. Changes in any of the individual components can affect the rest of the overall workings of the body. When hormones become imbalanced as a result of menopause (or whenever hormone fluctuations are likely to occur), the immune system can alter enough to make a woman more vulnerable to allergic conditions.

Treatments

Let's start with a heavy dose of common sense. Ask yourself, what can I do that'll make me feel better without causing side effects? We don't want to create bigger and different problems while trying to sort out your hay fever. *Lifestyle change* is the first strategy to consider. For instance, instead of immediately rushing to the chemist's for hay fever medications, try shutting the windows of the house to prevent pollen from entering or get an air filter that can drastically reduce allergenic particles in the air. Make sure there's an air/pollen filter installed in your car (newer models have this as standard). Look for good, strong wraparound eye protectors or sunglasses. Would you wear a face mask that filters pollen grains?

The following self-help tips are a guide to doing as much as you can without resorting to medicines. They were mentioned in Chapter 1 but there's no harm reinforcing them again.

- Avoid areas of lush grassland.
- Keep house and car windows closed during the peak pollen hours of late morning and late afternoon.
- Wear wraparound sunglasses to prevent pollen grains affecting the eyes.
- If you can, avoid being outdoors in the late morning and late afternoon.
- Don't smoke and keep away from smokers (passive smoking aggravates all allergies).
- Get someone else to mow the lawn or wear a face mask if you have to do it.
- Choose seaside breaks for holidays, as offshore breezes blow pollen away.
- Check TV, radio and newspapers for the next day's pollen count, and plan your schedule accordingly.
- Put a smear of Vaseline inside each nostril to ease the soreness and to capture pollen entering the nasal passages.
- Never sleep with the bedroom window open.
- Put used tea bags in the fridge. They make great soothing compresses to relieve swollen or puffy eyes.

Many menopausal women prefer to use natural remedies before turning to more orthodox treatments. Read the suggestions in

Chapter 11. Especially consider homeopathy, herbal supplements and acupuncture. If you do prefer natural remedies, bear in mind that your allergies are associated with hormonal changes and look for products that might restore balance. Here are a few immediate recommendations I have learned about from doctors who deal regularly with women troubled with allergy while going through the menopause.

Irene

Success has been reported by hay fever sufferers on a daily regime of Irene (see Chapter 11). A natural product without side effects, Irene is a blend of royal jelly, ginseng and echinacea. It is believed to act on the immune system, strengthening it for allergy challenge. Royal jelly has been used successfully in China for thousands of years to treat a large range of ailments. Its success is attributed to its balancing effect on the immune system. Ginseng has also been in use in Chinese herbal medicines for centuries, as has echinacea. Put together in a single and accessible product, the benefits of Irene are 'slow but steady'.

Omega-3 fatty acids

These may act to lower the amounts of inflammatory chemicals produced by the body after exposure to an allergen. Although additional research is needed, it appears that a diet high in omega-3 fatty acids may help decrease the incidence of hay fever in menopausal women.

Sanguinaria

This is a homeopathic preparation made from a herb that occurs naturally in the United States, Canada and India. It goes by the common name of bloodroot. Menopausal complaints that can be treated by sanguinaria include hay fever and asthma.

Practical tips

Here are some basic self-help tips for women experiencing the menopause. Use these suggestions in combination either with alternative remedies or standard medical therapies. Mix and match to suit your personality, the way the menopause is affecting you and the degree of hay fever symptoms you're experiencing.

Keep cool

Hot flushes and night sweats are the most common symptoms of the menopause. They're caused by a malfunction in the body's normal methods of temperature control. They can occur even before your periods have stopped, but are most common in the first year after your last period.

To ease hot flushes and night sweats:

● wear lighter clothing;
● keep your bedroom cool at night;
● do more exercise;
● try to reduce your stress levels;
● avoid potential triggers, such as spicy food, caffeine, smoking and alcohol.

Try to relax

Psychological symptoms can include feeling down, anxiety, irritability, mood swings, tiredness and lack of energy. However, this time in a woman's life can also be stressful due to parents' ageing and loss of independence, death of parents or relatives, divorce or 'empty nest syndrome' when children leave home. Therefore, it can be difficult to tell if your psychological symptoms are a direct result of the menopause.

The following tactics can help improve your mood:

● get plenty of rest;
● exercise regularly;
● do relaxation exercises such as yoga.

Sleep well

Restful sleep will help you cope with night sweats and other menopausal symptoms. Improve your sleep by:

● avoiding exercise within two hours of bedtime;
● going to bed at the same time every night.

Get some exercise

There's evidence that women who are active tend to suffer less from the symptoms of the menopause. Exercise is important not only for the relief of short-term symptoms but also to protect your body from heart disease and osteoporosis.

Exercise will help keep your bones and the muscles that support them strong. It will also increase your flexibility and mobility, which will in turn improve your balance.

The benefits of exercise in preventing bone loss and fractures are well known. The best activities are aerobic, sustained and regular. Brisk walking about three times a week is a cheap, easy and great way to start exercising.

Stop smoking

Women who smoke have an earlier menopause than non-smokers, have worse flushes and often don't respond as well to tablet forms of HRT. It's never too late to stop smoking.

Summary

Persisting hay fever can cause:

- a constantly blocked nose that may lead to sinusitis
- headaches
- aggressive sneezing
- runny nose (lots of tissues)
- itchy, red eyes
- damage to the surface of the eye from swellings behind the upper eyelids
- excessive tear production (watery eyes)
- diminished senses of taste and smell
- exhaustion
- asthma
- decreased ability to concentrate
- allergic irritability in children
- missed days at work or school
- reduced physical activity
- sleep apnoea.

However, by following the suggestions and advice in this book you or your child should be able to prevent suffering such ill-health.

References

Annesi-Maesano, I., 'Epidemiological evidence of the occurrence of rhinitis and sinusitis in asthmatics'. *Allergy* 54 (Suppl. 57), 1999, 7–13.

Aubier, M., Levy, J., Clerici, C., Neukirch, F., Herman, D., 'Different effects of nasal and bronchial glucocorticosteroid administration on bronchial hyperresponsiveness in patients with allergic rhinitis'. *American Review of Respiratory Disease* 146(1), July 1992, 122–6.

Bever, H. P. van, Potter, P. C., 'Making the allergic child happy: Treating more than symptoms'. *Clinical and Experimental Allergy Reviews* 6(1), Feb 2006, 6–9.

Braman, S. S., Barrows, A. A., DeCotiis, B. A., Settipane, G. A., Corrao, W. M., 'Airway hyperresponsiveness in allergic rhinitis: A risk factor for asthma'. *Chest* 91(5), May 1987, 671–4.

Ciprandi, G., Buscaglia, S., Pesce, G., Pronzato, C., Ricca, V., Parmiani, S., Bagnasco, M., Canonica, G. W., 'Minimal persistent inflammation is present at mucosal level in patients with asymptomatic rhinitis and mite allergy'. *Journal of Allergy and Clinical Immunology* 96(6 Pt 1), Dec 1995, 971–9.

Corren, J., 'The impact of allergic rhinitis on bronchial asthma'. *Journal of Allergy and Clinical Immunology* 101(2 Pt 2), Feb 1998, S352–S356.

Corren, J., Adinoff, A. D., Buchmeier, A. D., Irvin, C. G., 'Nasal beclomethasone prevents the seasonal increase in bronchial responsiveness in patients with allergic rhinitis and asthma'. *Journal of Allergy and Clinical Immunology* 90(2), Aug 1992, 250–6.

Denburg, J., 'The nose, the lung and the bone marrow in allergic inflammation'. *Allergy* 54 (Suppl. 57), 1999, 73–80.

Durham, S. R., Ying, S., Varney, V. A., Jacobson, M. R., Sudderick, R. M., Mackay, I. S., Kay, A. B., Hamid, Q. A., 'Grass pollen immunotherapy inhibits allergen-induced infiltration of CD4+ T lymphocytes and eosinophils in the nasal mucosa and increases the number of cells expressing messenger RNA for interferon-gamma'. *Journal of Allergy and Clinical Immunology* 97(6), June 1996, 1356–65.

Johnstone, D. E., Dutton, A., 'The value of hyposensitization therapy for bronchial asthma in children – a 14-year study'. *Pediatrics* 42(5), Nov 1968, 793–802.

Meltzer, E. O., 'Role for cysteinyl leukotriene receptor antagonist therapy in asthma and their potential role in allergic rhinitis based on the concept of "one linked airway disease"'. *Annals of Allergy, Asthma and Immunology* 84(2), Feb 2000, 176–87.

Ricca, V., Landi, M., Ferrero, P., Bairo, A., Tazzer, C., Canonica, G. W., Ciprandi, G., 'Minimal persistent inflammation is also present in patients with seasonal allergic rhinitis'. *Journal of Allergy and Clinical Immunology* 105(1 Pt 1), Jan 2000, 54–7.

Settipane, R. J., Hagy, G. W., Settipane, G. A., 'Long-term risk factors for developing asthma and allergic rhinitis: A 23-year follow-up study of college students'. *Allergy Proceedings* 15(1), Jan–Feb 1994, 21–5.

Simons, F. E., 'Allergic rhinobronchitis: The asthma–allergic rhinitis link'. *Journal of Allergy and Clinical Immunology* 104(3 Pt 1), Sep 1999, 534–40.

Spector, S. L., 'Overview of comorbid associations of allergic rhinitis'. *Journal of Allergy and Clinical Immunology* 99(2), Feb 1997, S773–S780.

Talbot, A. R., Herr, T. M. Parsons, D. S., 'Mucociliary clearance and buffered hypertonic saline solution'. *Laryngoscope* 107(4), 1997, 500–503.

'A teaching model for nasal irrigation'. *Journal of Allergy and Clinical Immunology* 11(1), 1998, 13–15.

Tomooka, L. T., Murphy, C., Davidson, T. M., 'Clinical study and literature review of nasal irrigation'. *Laryngoscope* 110(7), 2000, 1189–93.

Watson, W. T., Becker, A. B., Simons, F. E., 'Treatment of allergic rhinitis with intranasal corticosteroids in patients with mild asthma: Effect on lower airway responsiveness'. *Journal of Allergy and Clinical Immunology* 91(1 Pt 1), Jan 1993, 97–101.

Index